ATTITUDE-BASED SAFETY

Cultivating a Culture of Safety Through Positive Attitudes

Develop positive attitude, foster proactive practices, and create a resilient, accident-free environment.

by

Dr. Gurudas Bandyopadhyay

Visit: https://drgurudas.com

Unlock Your FREE GIFT Bundles

Claim your complimentary PDF Blueprint

Since you have embraced my book, ventured and have come up to this stage, I sense your eagerness to cultivate positive intentions and acquire further knowledge. As a gesture of gratitude, I extend this gift to you.

Visit here to get my Book for FREE:

https://winning-thinker-8854.ck.page/92cd3161e1

Over 130 pages book in pdf comprising 11 chapters.

Understand psychology behind incremental growth, need for celebrating small victories, understand power of mindset, and foster letting go through small wins.

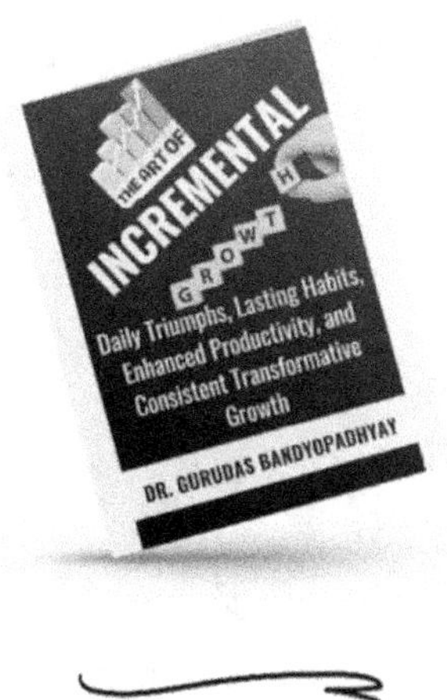

Objective of the book

Highlight the Role of Attitude in Safety: Emphasize the critical importance of attitude as the foundational element in achieving and maintaining safety in various settings.

Educate on Attitude Formation and Maintenance: Provide insights into how attitudes towards safety are formed and the strategies needed to maintain and reinforce positive attitudes.

Promote Positive Safety Behaviors: Offer practical guidance on translating positive safety attitudes into consistent, proactive safety behaviors.

Overcome Barriers to Safety Attitudes: Identify common barriers to adopting positive safety attitudes and provide effective solutions to overcome them.

Integrate Safety into Daily Practices: Demonstrate how to embed attitude-based safety into everyday routines, organizational culture, and community practices.

Measure and Sustain Safety Improvements: Present methods for assessing safety attitudes and behaviors, and strategies for sustaining long-term improvements in safety performance.

Empower Individuals and Leaders: Inspire and equip individuals and leaders with the tools and knowledge to take ownership of safety attitudes and drive cultural change within their organizations and communities.

Share Real-Life Examples and Research: Incorporate case studies, research reports, and real-life experiences to illustrate the principles and effectiveness of attitude-based safety.

Foster Continuous Improvement: Encourage an ongoing commitment to safety, emphasizing the importance of continuous learning, adaptation, and improvement in safety practices.

Create a Culture of Safety: Promote a holistic approach to safety that involves everyone—individuals, leaders, and communities—in building and maintaining a culture of safety awareness and responsibility.

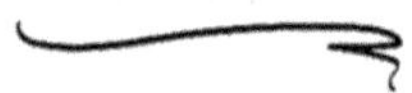

How to use the book

This book is designed to be a practical and comprehensive guide for understanding and implementing attitude-based safety in various aspects of life. Here's how you can make the most of it:

Start with the Introduction:

Begin by reading the introduction to grasp the foundational concepts of attitude-based safety and why it is crucial for personal, organizational, and social development.

Follow the Chapter Sequence:

The book is structured to build upon each chapter progressively. Start with Chapter 1 to understand the basics of attitude-based safety and continue sequentially to develop a deeper understanding and practical application.

Reflect on the Case Studies:

Each chapter includes case studies that illustrate real-life applications and lessons. Take the time to reflect on these examples and consider how they relate to your own experiences and environment.

Engage with the Sections and Sub-sections:

Each chapter is divided into sections and sub-sections that break down complex concepts into manageable parts. Use these divisions to focus on specific topics of interest or concern.

Utilize Practical Tips and Strategies:

The book provides numerous practical tips, strategies, and exercises. Actively engage with these suggestions to apply what you learn in real-world settings.

Incorporate Research and Evidence:

Pay attention to the research reports and evidence presented. These will help you understand the scientific basis behind the strategies and techniques discussed.

Participate in Self-assessment Activities:

Throughout the book, you'll find self-assessment activities designed to help you evaluate your current attitudes and behaviors towards safety. Use these tools to identify areas for improvement.

Implement Changes Gradually:

Implement the suggested changes gradually in your personal and professional life. Focus on one or two strategies at a time to ensure they are effectively integrated into your daily routine.

Share and Discuss with Others:

Share insights and discuss concepts with colleagues, family, and friends. Engaging others in conversation about attitude-based safety can foster a broader culture of safety awareness.

Refer as Needed:

Use the book as a reference guide. Return to specific chapters, sections, or tips as needed to reinforce your understanding and application of attitude-based safety principles.

Explore Additional Resources:

Check the "Additional Resources" section for further reading, exercises, and tools to continue your learning journey beyond this book.

Track Your Progress:

Regularly review and track your progress in adopting and maintaining positive safety attitudes and behaviors. Celebrate your successes and stay committed to continuous improvement.

By actively engaging with the content and applying the lessons learned, you will be well-equipped to foster a safer environment in both your personal and professional life.

Dedication

This book is dedicated to all those seeking to stay safe and to make
this world a safer and happier place to live in

Welcome

Dear Readers,

Welcome to "Attitude-Based Safety: Cultivating a Culture of Safety Through Positive Attitudes." In today's fast-paced and ever-evolving world, the importance of safety in our daily lives cannot be overstated. Whether at home, on the road, or in the workplace, our attitudes towards safety play a crucial role in preventing accidents and ensuring the well-being of ourselves and those around us.

This book is designed to guide you on a journey of self-discovery and empowerment, highlighting how a positive attitude towards safety can lead to profound changes in behavior and habits. By understanding and harnessing the power of attitude, we can create safer environments and foster a culture that prioritizes safety in every aspect of our lives.

Throughout this book, you will find insights drawn from years of research, case studies, and real-life experiences. These examples will illustrate the transformative impact that a positive safety attitude can have, not only on individual behavior but also on the collective mindset of organizations and communities.

We will explore practical strategies for developing and maintaining positive safety attitudes, overcoming barriers to change, and integrating safety into daily practices. Our goal is to provide you with the tools and knowledge needed to become a safety champion, leading by example and inspiring others to follow suit.

As you embark on this journey, remember that cultivating a culture of safety is a continuous process. It requires dedication, awareness, and a commitment to lifelong learning. Together, we can make a difference and achieve the ultimate goal of zero accidents and injuries.

Thank you for joining us in this important endeavor. Let's work together to create a safer, healthier, and more resilient world.

Sincerely,

Dr. Gurudas Bandyopadhyay

Preface

In an era where advancements in technology and industrial growth are at their peak, the emphasis on safety has never been more critical. The world around us is constantly changing, bringing about new challenges and risks. Despite these changes, one factor remains a constant pillar in ensuring our well-being: attitude.

"Attitude-Based Safety: Cultivating a Culture of Safety Through Positive Attitudes" is born out of a profound understanding that the foundation of all safety measures lies in the attitudes we hold. Our attitudes shape our behaviors, which in turn, become our habits. It is these habits that ultimately define the safety standards we uphold in our personal lives, workplaces, and communities.

The inspiration to write this book stems from my extensive experience spanning various sectors, including heavy engineering, petrochemicals, and construction. Throughout my career, I have witnessed firsthand the transformative power of a positive safety attitude. From reducing workplace accidents to fostering a culture of proactive safety measures, the impact is undeniable. I have gathered valuable experience in safety observation tours, accident investigation and post-accident interviews with the victims and their near and dear ones, which

I want to share so that people take better care for their safety and can contribute a lot for their family, organization and the society.

The need for this book is both urgent and significant. Every day, countless accidents occur due to carelessness and a lack of safety awareness. These incidents are not just statistics; they are personal tragedies that affect families, organizations, and societies at large. By addressing the core of these issues—our attitudes—we can create a ripple effect that enhances safety across all levels.

This book is intended for everyone who values safety, whether you are an individual seeking to protect yourself and your loved ones, a leader striving to cultivate a safe working environment, or a community member dedicated to fostering a culture of safety. It provides practical strategies, real-life examples, and actionable insights designed to help you develop and sustain positive safety attitudes.

Safety is not merely a set of rules to follow; it is a mindset, a way of life. By understanding the importance of attitude, we can drive significant improvements in safety practices and create environments where everyone feels secure and protected. This book aims to equip you with the knowledge and tools to embark on this journey of transformation.

Thank you for choosing to explore this crucial topic. Together, we can make a lasting impact and move towards a safer, healthier, and more resilient world.

Table of Contents

Introduction

A short story from personal experiences

As the early morning light gently painted the horizon, I embarked on my routine duty rounds, unaware of the life-altering events that would unfold. Within moments, a frantic call shattered the tranquility of the day - a worker had fallen from a height of 15 feet while descending from his duties. Reacting swiftly, I, as Safety Team Leader, along with my team and representatives from the concerned department, rushed to the scene.

Upon arrival, the grim reality became apparent. The victim, through a series of unfortunate lapses in judgment, had neglected to don his Personal Protective Equipment (PPE) and embarked on his descent with an empty stomach, battling a burgeoning headache in silence. These critical oversights would soon culminate in a harrowing injury to his head, sending shockwaves through the entire workforce nearby.

Swift action was taken, and the injured worker was promptly transported to the nearest hospital, where his life hung in the balance. Miraculously, he survived, but the incident left an indelible mark, serving as a stark reminder of the grave consequences of negative safety attitude and neglecting self-care.

Reflecting on this striking experience, one cannot help but draw invaluable lessons. Adherence to safety measures, such as wearing PPE and adhering to Standard Operating

Procedures (SOPs), is not merely a matter of compliance - it's a lifeline, safeguarding against unforeseen hazards that lurk within the workplace.

Furthermore, the incident underscores the importance of prioritizing personal well-being. Concealing ailments, however trivial they may seem, joining duty empty stomach can have catastrophic repercussions, not only for oneself but for the loved ones who depend on him or her. True security lies not in fleeting shortcuts but in steadfast commitment to long-term safety and prosperity.

As we navigate the complexities of our daily lives, let us heed the lessons learned from this cautionary tale. Let us show our positive attitude to stay safe, pledge to embrace safety as a guiding principle, safeguarding not only our present but our collective future as well.

INTRODUCTION TO THE CONCEPT OF ATTITUDE FOR ACCIDENT PREVENTION

Whether at home, on the road, or in the workplace, in the field of safety, the concept of attitude plays a pivotal role in accident prevention. Understanding and harnessing the power of attitude can lead to significant improvements in safety outcomes. Here's a deeper dive into this crucial concept:

Attitude in Safety Context

Attitude, in the context of safety, refers to an individual's settled way of thinking or feeling about safety-related matters, which often influences their behavior and decision-making. It encompasses a range of mental states, including beliefs, feelings, and values about safety practices and risk perception.

The Role of Attitude in Accident Prevention

Influence on Behavior:

Attitude significantly influences behavior. A positive attitude towards safety can lead to proactive safety behaviors, such as consistently wearing protective equipment, adhering to safety protocols, and staying vigilant for potential hazards. Conversely, a negative attitude can result in negligence, risk-taking, and complacency, increasing the likelihood of accidents.

Perception of Risks:

Individuals with a positive safety attitude are more likely to perceive risks accurately and take appropriate precautions. They understand the potential consequences of unsafe actions and are motivated to avoid risky behaviors. Those with a dismissive attitude towards safety may underestimate risks and overlook necessary precautions.

Commitment to Safety:

A positive safety attitude fosters a commitment to maintaining a safe environment. This commitment is reflected in an individual's willingness to participate in safety training, report hazards, and comply with safety regulations. It also encourages the adoption of continuous improvement practices, leading to safer conditions over time.

WHY ATTITUDE IS CRUCIAL FOR ACCIDENT PREVENTION

Attitude as a precursor to action:

Attitude serves as the precursor to action. The way individuals think and feel about safety directly impacts their actions. By cultivating a positive safety attitude, organizations and individuals can ensure that safety becomes a priority and a habitual practice.

Cultural impact:

Attitude extends beyond the individual level and contributes to the overall safety culture of an organization or community. A collective positive attitude towards safety can create an environment where safety is ingrained in every aspect of operations, leading to widespread adherence to safe practices and a reduction in accidents.

Long-term benefits:

Fostering a positive safety attitude can lead to long-term benefits, such as reduced accident rates, lower healthcare costs, and improved employee morale and productivity. It also enhances the reputation of organizations, making them more attractive to clients, customers, and potential employees.

Education and Training:

Regular education and training sessions can help individuals understand the importance of safety and develop the knowledge needed to maintain a positive attitude towards it. These sessions should include both theoretical knowledge and practical applications.

Leadership and Role Modeling:

Leaders play a critical role in shaping attitudes. By modeling positive safety behaviors and attitudes, leaders can influence their teams to adopt similar practices. Leadership commitment to safety sends a strong message about its importance.

Communication and Engagement:

Open and effective communication about safety issues, successes, and challenges helps keep safety at the forefront of everyone's mind. Engaging employees in safety initiatives and decision-making processes also fosters a sense of ownership and accountability.

Recognition and Rewards:

Recognizing and rewarding individuals and teams for demonstrating positive

HOW ATTITUDE FORM THE FOUNDATION TO REACH ZERO
UNSAFE BEHAVIOR

Achieving zero unsafe behavior is an ambitious yet critical goal for any safety-focused organization or community. At the heart of this endeavor lies the concept of attitude. Attitude serves as the bedrock upon which safe behaviors are built and maintained. Here's a detailed explanation of how a positive attitude forms the foundation to reach zero unsafe behavior:

Understanding the Link Between Attitude and Behavior

Attitude influences Perception:

A positive safety attitude shapes how individuals perceive their environment and the potential risks within it. When safety is viewed as a priority, individuals are more likely to recognize and acknowledge hazards, leading to more cautious and responsible behavior.

Attitude drives Motivation:

A strong, positive attitude towards safety motivates individuals to engage in safe practices consistently. This intrinsic motivation ensures that safety protocols are followed not just out of obligation, but because individuals believe in their importance and are committed to maintaining a safe environment.

Attitude shapes Habits:

When individuals hold a positive attitude towards safety, it becomes easier to develop and sustain safe habits. These habits, formed through repeated safe behaviors, become second nature, reducing the likelihood of unsafe actions over time.

COMPONENTS OF A POSITIVE SAFETY ATTITUDE

Awareness:

Awareness of the importance of safety and the potential consequence of unsafe behavior is the first step in developing a positive safety attitude. This awareness drives individuals to prioritize safety in their daily activities.

Responsibility:

A positive attitude towards safety involves taking personal responsibility for one's own safety and the safety of others. This sense of responsibility encourages proactive measures to prevent accidents and unsafe conditions.

Commitment:

Commitment to safety means consistently striving to improve safety practices and behaviors. This commitment often leads to continuous learning and adaptation, essential for maintaining high safety standards.

Strategies to Cultivate a Positive Safety Attitude

Education and Training:

Regular education and training programs help individuals understand the importance of safety and how their attitudes impact behavior. These programs should emphasize the connection between attitude and safety outcomes.

Leadership Example:

Leaders play a crucial role in shaping attitudes. When leaders demonstrate a strong commitment to safety through their actions and decisions, it sets a powerful example for others to follow.

Positive Reinforcement:

Recognizing and rewarding safe behaviors reinforces the value of a positive safety attitude. Positive reinforcement can come in many forms, such as praise, awards, or incentives, and helps to embed safety into the organizational culture.

Creating a Safety Culture Through Positive Attitude

Organizational Values:

Integrating safety into the core values of an organization ensures that safety attitudes are prioritized at every level. When safety is part of the organizational ethos, it becomes a shared responsibility.

Communication:

Open and effective communication about safety issues, successes, and challenges helps reinforce a positive safety attitude. Regular safety meetings, updates, and discussions keep safety top of mind for everyone.

Engagement and Involvement:

Involving employees in safety initiatives and decision-making processes fosters a sense of ownership and accountability. Engaged employees are more likely to develop and maintain positive attitudes towards safety.

IMPACT OF POSITIVE SAFETY ATTITUDE ON BEHAVIOR

Reduction in Unsafe Acts:

A positive safety attitude directly reduces the frequency of unsafe acts. Individuals with a strong safety mindset are less likely to take unnecessary risks or ignore safety protocols.

Enhanced Reporting and Feedback:

A positive attitude towards safety encourages open reporting of hazards, near-misses, and unsafe conditions. This openness leads to timely interventions and continuous improvement in safety practices.

Sustainable Safety Practices:

Sustaining zero unsafe behaviors requires long-term commitment and consistent effort. A positive safety attitude ensures that safe behaviors are not just a temporary focus but are embedded in the daily routines and practices of individuals and organizations.

Attitude is the foundation upon which zero unsafe behavior is built. By fostering a positive safety attitude, individuals and organizations can create an environment where safe practices are the norm, not the exception. This foundational shift in mindset and behavior is crucial for achieving and maintaining high safety standards, ultimately leading to a safer and more productive environment for all.

Setting the stage for readers to embark on a journey of self-discovery and empowerment.

Welcome, dear reader, to a transformative journey towards self-discovery and empowerment in the realm of safety. As you embark on this path, you are not merely a passive observer but an active participant in shaping your safety mindset and behaviors.

Within the pages of this book, you will encounter insights, strategies, and reflections that will challenge your existing perceptions and inspire profound shifts in your approach to safety. But this journey is not just about acquiring knowledge; it's about embracing a new way of thinking and being—a way that empowers you to take control of your safety and well-being.

As you delve deeper into the concepts presented here, you will uncover layers of understanding about the intricate interplay between attitude, behavior, and safety outcomes. You will confront barriers and limitations that may have held you back in the past and discover the untapped potential within yourself to create a safer and more resilient future.

But remember, this journey is not without its challenges. It requires courage to confront ingrained beliefs and habits, and dedication to implement lasting change.

Yet, with each step forward, you will find yourself growing stronger, more confident, and more capable of navigating the complexities of the safety landscape.

So, I invite you to approach this journey with an open mind and a willing heart. Embrace the opportunity to explore new perspectives, engage in self-reflection, and chart a course towards a safer, more empowered future.

Together, let us embark on this journey of self-discovery and empowerment, knowing that the destination—zero unsafe behavior—is within our reach.

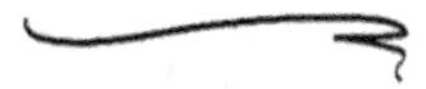

Chapter 1: Understanding Attitude-Based Safety

Safety is not a gadget but a state of mind

- Eleanor Everet

Attitude-Based Safety (ABS) is a proactive approach to safety management that emphasizes the pivotal role of attitudes in shaping behaviors and driving safety outcomes. At its core, ABS recognizes that attitudes serve as powerful predictors of behavior: positive attitudes tend to lead to safe actions, while negative attitudes can increase the likelihood of risky behaviors and accidents.

The concept of ABS operates on the fundamental understanding that attitudes are not fixed, but rather malleable and influenced by various factors such as past experiences, social norms, organizational culture, and individual perceptions. Therefore, by intentionally cultivating positive attitudes towards safety, organizations and individuals can create an environment where safe actions are not only encouraged but become ingrained in the organizational culture and individual mindset.

ABS acknowledges that safety is not just a set of rules or procedures to be followed but is deeply rooted in individual beliefs, values, and motivations. By focusing on fostering positive safety attitudes, ABS seeks to:

Initiate Safe Actions: Positive safety attitudes serve as catalysts for initiating safe actions. When individuals possess a strong belief in the importance of safety and a commitment to practicing safe behaviors, they are more likely to proactively identify and mitigate risks, follow safety protocols, and prioritize safety in their decision-making processes.

Drive Continuous Improvement: ABS encourages a culture of continuous improvement by promoting a growth mindset towards safety. Individuals with positive safety attitudes are more open to feedback, learning, and adapting their behaviors based on new information or experiences. This mindset fosters innovation, collaboration, and a willingness to embrace change for the sake of enhancing safety outcomes.

Mitigate Risk and Prevent Accidents: By instilling a culture of safety consciousness and vigilance, ABS helps organizations mitigate risks and prevent accidents before they occur. When individuals possess positive safety attitudes, they are more likely to anticipate potential hazards, intervene in unsafe situations, and take proactive measures to prevent accidents and injuries.

Promote Organizational Resilience: A workforce with positive safety attitudes is better equipped to navigate challenges, setbacks, and unforeseen circumstances. In times of crisis or emergency, individuals who prioritize safety and possess a resilient mindset are more likely to remain calm, make informed decisions, and effectively respond to hazards, thereby minimizing the impact of adverse events on organizational performance and reputation.

In essence, Attitude-Based Safety underscores the transformative power of attitudes in driving safe actions, fostering a culture of safety, and ultimately, safeguarding the well-being of individuals and organizations. By recognizing the inherent connection between attitudes and behaviors, ABS empowers individuals to take ownership of their safety mindset and become proactive agents of change in creating safer workplaces and communities.

1.1 THE POWER OF ATTITUDE IN SAFETY

1.1.1 Recognizing the Impact: Explore real-life examples where positive attitudes have led to safer work environments and reduced accidents.

Real-life examples abound where positive attitudes have been instrumental in fostering safer work environments and reducing accidents. Here are a few illustrative scenarios:

Safety Leadership and Empowerment: In a manufacturing facility, a supervisor consistently demonstrates a positive attitude towards safety by prioritizing safety discussions, conducting regular safety audits, and actively engaging employees in safety initiatives. Inspired by their supervisor's commitment to safety, employees feel empowered to voice safety concerns, suggest improvements, and proactively address hazards. As a result, the facility experiences a significant reduction in accidents and near-misses, leading to a safer and more productive work environment.

Safety Culture Transformation: A construction company undergoes a safety culture transformation initiative aimed at instilling a positive safety attitude among its workforces. Through targeted training, communication campaigns, and leadership reinforcement, employees begin to internalize the importance of safety and embrace safety as a core value. As attitudes shift towards a collective commitment to safety, workers become more vigilant, proactive, and accountable for their safety and the safety of their peers. This cultural shift results in a dramatic decrease in accidents, injuries, and lost workdays, demonstrating the tangible impact of positive safety attitudes on overall safety performance.

Employee Engagement and Ownership: In a healthcare setting, nurses and medical staff exhibit a positive safety attitude by actively participating in safety committees, conducting safety hurdles, and implementing safety best practices. Their collective commitment to safety fosters a culture of transparency, collaboration, and continuous improvement, where staff feel empowered to identify and address safety concerns in real-time. This proactive approach to safety leads to enhanced patient outcomes, reduced medical errors, and a safer healthcare environment for both patients and staff.

Safety Innovation and Creativity: In an industrial setting, a group of frontline workers with a positive safety attitude collaborates to develop innovative safety solutions to address ergonomic hazards and repetitive motion injuries. Drawing on their collective knowledge and creativity, they design and implement new equipment modifications and work processes that minimize ergonomic risks and improve worker comfort and safety. Their proactive approach to safety not only reduces the incidence of workplace injuries but also fosters a culture of innovation and continuous improvement across the organization.

These real-life examples demonstrate the profound impact of positive safety attitudes on creating safer work environments, preventing accidents, and enhancing overall safety performance. By recognizing and celebrating the contributions of individuals with positive safety attitudes, organizations can inspire others to embrace safety as a shared responsibility and drive meaningful change towards a safer future.

1.1.2 Understanding Psychological Mechanisms: Delve into the cognitive and emotional processes that underpin attitudes and their influence on safety behaviors.

Exploring the cognitive and emotional processes that underpin attitudes is essential for understanding how they influence safety behaviors. Here's an exploration of the psychological mechanisms at play:

Cognitive Processes: Attitudes are formed and shaped through cognitive processes such as perception, judgment, and belief systems. Individuals interpret safety-related information based on their past experiences, knowledge, and cognitive biases. For example, someone who has had positive experiences with safety protocols may develop a favorable attitude towards safety, while someone who has encountered obstacles or resistance may harbor negative attitudes. Cognitive appraisal theory suggests that individuals evaluate safety-related stimuli based on their perceived relevance, significance, and potential consequences, which in turn influence their attitudes and subsequent behaviors.

Emotional Processes: Emotions play a significant role in shaping attitudes towards safety. Positive emotions such as enthusiasm, confidence, and trust can enhance individuals' receptivity to safety messages and motivate them to engage in safe behaviors. Conversely, negative emotions such as fear, anxiety, and frustration can evoke defensive reactions or resistance to safety initiatives. The affective forecasting theory suggests that individuals' attitudes and behaviors are influenced by their anticipated emotional outcomes, leading them to avoid or embrace safety-related activities based on their anticipated emotional responses.

Social Processes: Attitudes are also influenced by social factors such as social norms, peer pressure, and group dynamics. Social identity theory posits that individuals derive a sense of identity and belonging from their affiliation with social groups and may adopt the attitudes and behaviors endorsed by their group members. Therefore, organizational culture, leadership behavior, and peer interactions play a critical role in shaping individuals' attitudes towards safety. For example, positive safety role models and supportive social networks can reinforce positive safety attitudes, while negative social influences or group norms that prioritize productivity over safety may undermine safety efforts.

Motivational Processes: Motivation is another key psychological mechanism that influences attitudes and behaviors towards safety. Self-determination theory suggests that individuals are motivated by intrinsic factors such as autonomy, competence, and relatedness, as well as extrinsic factors such as rewards, recognition, and consequences. Therefore, organizations can enhance individuals' motivation to engage in safe behaviors by providing meaningful feedback, opportunities for skill development, and a supportive work environment that fosters a sense of belonging and purpose.

By understanding these psychological mechanisms, organizations can design more effective safety interventions and communication strategies that appeal to individuals' cognitive, emotional, social, and motivational needs. By addressing the underlying drivers of attitudes towards safety, organizations can create a culture of safety where individuals feel empowered, motivated, and committed to prioritizing safety in their actions and decisions.

1.1.3 Leveraging Attitudes for Change: Provide actionable strategies for harnessing the power of positive attitudes to drive safety improvements.

Harnessing the power of positive attitudes is essential for driving safety improvements within organizations. Here are actionable strategies for leveraging attitudes for change:

Leadership Commitment: Leadership plays a crucial role in shaping organizational culture and driving safety improvements. Leaders should demonstrate a visible commitment to safety by actively promoting and endorsing positive safety attitudes. This can be achieved through regular communication, setting clear safety expectations, leading by example, and allocating resources to support safety initiatives.

Education and Training: Providing comprehensive safety education and training programs is essential for instilling positive safety attitudes among employees. Training should not only focus on technical skills and compliance but also emphasize the importance of safety culture, risk awareness, and individual responsibility. Interactive and engaging training methods, such as scenario-based simulations, role-playing exercises, and peer-to-peer learning, can effectively reinforce positive safety attitudes.

Promoting Open Communication: Creating a culture of open communication where employees feel comfortable sharing safety concerns, reporting near-misses, and providing feedback is crucial for driving safety improvements.

Employers should establish multiple channels for communication, such as safety suggestion boxes, anonymous reporting systems, and regular safety meetings, to encourage employee engagement and participation in safety initiatives.

Empowering Employee Involvement: Empowering employees to actively participate in safety decision-making and problem-solving processes can foster a sense of ownership and accountability for safety outcomes.

Employers should involve frontline workers in safety committees, hazard identification teams, and safety improvement projects, allowing them to contribute their expertise, insights, and ideas for enhancing safety practices.

Recognition and Reward Systems: Implementing recognition and reward systems that reinforce positive safety attitudes and behaviors can motivate employees to prioritize safety in their daily activities.

Recognizing individuals and teams for their contributions to safety, whether through formal awards, certificates of appreciation, or public acknowledgment, sends a powerful message that safety is valued and appreciated within the organization.

Continuous Improvement: Foster a culture of continuous improvement by encouraging employees to identify areas for safety enhancement and implement innovative solutions. Employers should establish mechanisms for soliciting employee suggestions, conducting safety audits, and evaluating the effectiveness of safety initiatives to identify opportunities for improvement and address emerging safety challenges proactively.

By leveraging these strategies to harness the power of positive attitudes, organizations can create a culture of safety where safety is ingrained in the organizational DNA, and employees are empowered and motivated to prioritize safety in everything they do.

Ultimately, this proactive approach to safety can drive meaningful improvements in safety performance, reduce accidents and injuries, and create safer and healthier workplaces for all employees.

1.2 ATTITUDE FORMATION AND MAINTENANCE

1.2.1 Tracing Origins: Discuss how past experiences, social influences, and organizational culture contribute to the formation of attitudes towards safety.

Understanding the origins of attitudes towards safety is essential for effectively addressing them within organizations. Here's a discussion on how past experiences, social influences, and organizational culture contribute to attitude formation and maintenance:

Past Experiences: Individuals' past experiences shape their attitudes towards safety by influencing their perceptions of risk, trust in safety protocols, and beliefs about their ability to control their safety outcomes. Positive experiences, such as receiving adequate safety training, witnessing safety protocols in action, or experiencing successful hazard mitigations, can foster a sense of confidence and trust in safety measures. Conversely, negative experiences, such as accidents, near-misses, or ineffective safety procedures, can instill fear, skepticism, or complacency towards safety efforts. Therefore, organizations must acknowledge the impact of past experiences on attitudes and provide opportunities for individuals to reflect on and learn from their experiences to promote positive safety attitudes.

Social Influences: Social influences, including peer pressure, group norms, and leadership behavior, significantly impact attitudes towards safety within organizations. Individuals often conform to the attitudes and behaviors of their social groups, seeking acceptance and validation from their peers and leaders. Therefore, positive safety attitudes modeled by influential leaders and respected peers can serve as powerful drivers for shaping collective safety attitudes within teams and departments. Conversely, negative social influences, such as resistance to safety initiatives or peer pressure to prioritize productivity over safety, can undermine efforts to promote positive safety attitudes. Organizations must foster a culture of safety that encourages open communication, mutual support, and collective accountability to counteract negative social influences and promote positive safety attitudes.

Organizational Culture: Organizational culture plays a pivotal role in shaping attitudes towards safety by establishing norms, values, and expectations related to safety within the workplace. A safety-oriented culture, characterized by leadership commitment, employee empowerment, and a focus on continuous improvement, cultivates positive safety attitudes among employees. Conversely, a culture that prioritizes productivity over safety, tolerates unsafe behaviors, or lacks accountability for safety outcomes can foster negative safety attitudes and undermine safety efforts. Therefore, organizations must assess and cultivate a positive safety culture that aligns with their values and objectives, leveraging leadership support, employee involvement, and organizational policies to reinforce positive safety attitudes and behaviors.

By understanding how past experiences, social influences, and organizational culture contribute to attitude formation and maintenance, organizations can develop targeted interventions and initiatives to promote positive safety attitudes among employees. By addressing these underlying factors, organizations can create a safer and healthier workplace culture where safety is valued, prioritized, and embraced by all employees.

1.2.2 Nurturing Attitudes Over Time: Offer practical tips for maintaining and reinforcing positive safety attitudes through ongoing education, communication, and reinforcement.

Maintaining and reinforcing positive safety attitudes over time is essential for creating a sustainable culture of safety within organizations. Here are some practical tips for nurturing attitudes towards safety:

Ongoing Education and Training: Provide regular safety education and training sessions to keep employees informed about safety protocols, procedures, and best practices. Offer refresher courses, toolbox talks, and safety seminars to reinforce key safety messages and address emerging safety concerns. Use a variety of training methods, such as e-learning modules, hands-on simulations, and group discussions, to cater to different learning styles and preferences.

Effective Communication: Foster open and transparent communication channels to facilitate dialogue about safety issues, concerns, and successes. Encourage employees to share their thoughts, experiences, and suggestions for improving safety practices. Use multiple communication channels, such as safety newsletters, bulletin boards, and digital platforms, to disseminate safety-related information and updates. Ensure that safety messages are clear, concise, and accessible to all employees, regardless of their role or level within the organization.

Positive Reinforcement: Recognize and reward positive safety attitudes and behaviors to reinforce their importance and encourage continued compliance. Implement a formal recognition program that acknowledges individuals and teams for their contributions to safety, such as safety awards, incentive programs, or public commendations. Provide constructive feedback and encouragement to employees who demonstrate a commitment to safety, highlighting specific examples of safe behaviors and their positive impact on workplace safety.

Lead by Example: Leadership plays a critical role in setting the tone for safety culture within an organization. Leaders should demonstrate a visible commitment to safety by adhering to safety protocols, actively participating in safety initiatives, and prioritizing safety in decision-making processes. Encourage leaders to engage with employees on safety-related matters, solicit their input and feedback, and model safe behaviors in their day-to-day activities. By leading by example, leaders can inspire trust, confidence, and accountability in safety throughout the organization.

Employee Empowerment: Empower employees to take ownership of their safety and the safety of their colleagues by involving them in safety-related decision-making processes. Encourage employees to identify hazards, report near misses, and suggest improvements to safety procedures. Provide opportunities for employees to participate in safety committees, task forces, and improvement projects, allowing them to contribute their expertise and insights to enhance safety practices. Empower frontline workers to intervene in unsafe situations and advocate for safety improvements without fear of reprisal or retribution.

By implementing these practical tips for maintaining and reinforcing positive safety attitudes, organizations can create a culture of safety that is ingrained in the daily practices and behaviors of all employees. By nurturing attitudes towards safety over time, organizations can drive continuous improvement in safety performance, reduce accidents and injuries, and create safer and healthier workplaces for all employees.

1.2.3 Addressing Negativity: Explore techniques for identifying and addressing negative attitudes towards safety, including open dialogue, empathy, and support.

Addressing negative attitudes towards safety is crucial for promoting a positive safety culture within organizations. Here are some techniques for identifying and addressing negativity:

Open Dialogue: Foster open and honest communication channels where employees feel comfortable expressing their concerns, frustrations, and doubts about safety. Encourage managers and supervisors to hold regular safety meetings or toolbox talks where employees can voice their opinions, share their experiences, and raise any safety-related issues they may encounter. Create a safe space for employees to ask questions, seek clarification, and provide feedback on safety practices and procedures.

Empathy: Demonstrate empathy and understanding towards employees who express negative attitudes towards safety. Acknowledge their concerns and listen actively to their perspectives without judgment or criticism. Validate their experiences and emotions and reassure them that their safety is a top priority for the organization. Empathetic responses can help build trust and rapport with employees, making them feel valued and supported in their efforts to address safety concerns.

Support: Provide support and resources to help employees overcome negative attitudes towards safety and develop a more positive outlook. Offer counseling services, employee assistance programs, or peer support groups for employees who may be struggling with safety-related anxiety, stress, or trauma. Provide access to additional training, mentoring, or coaching to help employees improve their understanding of safety principles and build confidence in their ability to work safely. By offering practical support and guidance, organizations can empower employees to overcome negativity and embrace a culture of safety.

Education and Awareness: Educate employees about the consequences of negative attitudes towards safety and the importance of adopting a positive mindset for accident prevention. Raise awareness about the impact of negative attitudes on workplace safety, productivity, and employee well-being through training sessions, safety campaigns, or informational materials. Highlight real-life examples and case studies where negative attitudes have led to accidents or near misses, emphasizing the importance of vigilance, responsibility, and teamwork in maintaining a safe work environment.

Promote a Culture of Accountability: Encourage accountability for safety at all levels of the organization by holding individuals responsible for their attitudes and behaviors towards safety. Establish clear expectations for safety performance and conduct regular assessments to monitor compliance and identify areas for improvement. Recognize and reward employees who demonstrate positive safety attitudes and behaviors, while addressing negative behaviors through corrective action and coaching. By promoting a culture of accountability, organizations can create a sense of shared responsibility for safety and discourage negative attitudes that may compromise workplace safety.

By utilizing these techniques for identifying and addressing negative attitudes towards safety, organizations can create a supportive environment where employees feel empowered to overcome challenges, embrace positive attitudes, and work together towards a common goal of creating a safer and healthier workplace.

1.3 ATTITUDE AS THE CORE FACTOR

1.3.1 Integrating Attitude into Safety Practices: Illustrate how attitudes serve as the cornerstone of effective safety programs and initiatives.

Integrating attitude into safety practices is essential for creating a culture of safety within organizations. Here's how attitudes serve as the cornerstone of effective safety programs and initiatives:

Setting the Tone: Attitudes towards safety set the tone for organizational safety culture. When employees prioritize safety and demonstrate positive safety attitudes, it signals a collective commitment to workplace safety. Leaders play a crucial role in modeling positive safety attitudes and behaviors, influencing the attitudes of their teams and shaping the overall safety climate within the organization.

Driving Behavior: Attitudes towards safety influence employee behavior and decision-making processes. Positive safety attitudes promote a proactive approach to safety, encouraging employees to actively identify hazards, follow safety protocols, and intervene in unsafe situations. By emphasizing the importance of safety attitudes, organizations can empower employees to take ownership of their safety and the safety of their colleagues, leading to safer work practices and reduced accident rates.

Embedding Safety in Organizational Culture: Safety attitudes are embedded within the fabric of organizational culture, guiding norms, values, and expectations related to safety. When safety attitudes align with organizational values and objectives, it creates a supportive environment where safety is prioritized in all aspects of operations. Integrating safety attitudes into organizational culture involves fostering open communication, promoting accountability, and recognizing and rewarding positive safety behaviors.

Enhancing Risk Awareness: Positive safety attitudes enhance risk awareness among employees, enabling them to recognize potential hazards and take appropriate precautions to mitigate risks. When employees possess a safety-conscious mindset, they are more likely to anticipate, identify, and respond to safety threats proactively. By integrating safety attitudes into risk management processes, organizations can improve hazard identification, risk assessment, and risk control measures, ultimately reducing the likelihood of accidents and injuries.

Promoting Continuous Improvement: Safety attitudes drive continuous improvement in safety performance by encouraging feedback, learning, and adaptation. When employees embrace a growth mindset towards safety, they are more receptive to feedback, eager to learn from mistakes, and committed to ongoing improvement. By fostering a culture of continuous improvement, organizations can adapt to changing safety challenges, implement innovative solutions, and strive towards achieving excellence in safety performance.

In summary, integrating attitude into safety practices is essential for creating a culture of safety where positive safety attitudes serve as the foundation for effective safety programs and initiatives. By recognizing the pivotal role of attitudes in shaping safety outcomes, organizations can cultivate a safety-conscious mindset among employees, drive positive safety behaviors, and create safer and healthier work environments for all.

1.3.2 Aligning Organizational Values: Discuss the importance of aligning organizational values and objectives with a commitment to fostering positive safety attitudes.

Aligning organizational values and objectives with a commitment to fostering positive safety attitudes is crucial for creating a strong safety culture within an organization. Here's why it's important:

Cultural Consistency: When organizational values and objectives prioritize safety, it sends a clear message to employees that safety is a top priority. This consistency helps to reinforce the importance of safety in all aspects of the organization's operations, from strategic decision-making to daily work practices.

Employee Engagement: Aligning organizational values with safety fosters greater employee engagement and buy-in to safety initiatives. When employees see that safety is valued by leadership and integrated into the organization's mission and values, they are more likely to actively participate in safety programs, follow safety procedures, and take ownership of safety in their work areas.

Trust and Credibility: Organizations that prioritize safety in their values and objectives build trust and credibility with employees, customers, and other stakeholders. By demonstrating a commitment to safety, organizations show that they care about the well-being of their employees and are dedicated to providing a safe and healthy work environment. This enhances the organization's reputation and helps to attract and retain top talent.

Consistent Decision-Making: When safety is aligned with organizational values, it becomes a guiding principle in decision-making processes at all levels of the organization. Leaders and employees alike are more likely to consider safety implications when making decisions about processes, procedures, and resource allocation. This leads to more informed and responsible decision-making that prioritizes safety outcomes.

Continuous Improvement: Organizational values that emphasize safety encourage a culture of continuous improvement in safety performance. When safety is embedded in the organization's values and objectives, employees are motivated to seek out opportunities for improvement, identify hazards, and implement proactive safety measures. This continuous improvement mindset drives ongoing progress towards achieving safety goals and objectives.

In summary, aligning organizational values and objectives with a commitment to fostering positive safety attitudes is essential for creating a culture of safety where safety is ingrained in the organization's DNA. By prioritizing safety in values and objectives, organizations can engage employees, build trust, make consistent decisions, and drive continuous improvement in safety performance.

1.3.3 Empowering Individuals: Provide guidance on empowering individuals at all levels of the organization to take ownership of their attitudes towards safety and drive positive change.

Empowering individuals at all levels of the organization to take ownership of their attitudes towards safety is crucial for driving positive change and fostering a culture of safety. Here's how organizations can provide guidance on empowering individuals:

Education and Training: Offer comprehensive education and training programs to equip individuals with the knowledge and skills they need to understand the importance of safety attitudes and behaviors. Provide training on hazard recognition, risk assessment, safety procedures, and effective communication to empower individuals to make informed decisions and take proactive steps to enhance safety.

Encourage Open Communication: Create an environment where individuals feel comfortable expressing their concerns, ideas, and suggestions related to safety. Encourage open dialogue between employees and management and provide channels for feedback and reporting of safety issues. By fostering a culture of open communication, individuals are empowered to voice their opinions and contribute to safety improvement efforts.

Promote Leadership Support: Ensure that leaders at all levels of the organization actively demonstrate their commitment to safety and provide support and encouragement to individuals. Leaders should lead by example by adhering to safety protocols, promoting safety initiatives, and recognizing and rewarding positive safety attitudes and behaviors. By demonstrating leadership support for safety, individuals are motivated to prioritize safety in their actions and decisions.

Empowerment through Responsibility: Delegate responsibility for safety to individuals across the organization and empower them to take ownership of safety in their respective roles. Provide individuals with the authority to implement safety improvements, address safety concerns, and intervene in unsafe situations. By giving individuals, a sense of ownership and accountability for safety, they are more likely to proactively identify and address safety issues in their work areas.

Provide Resources and Support: Ensure that individuals have access to the resources and support they need to maintain positive safety attitudes and behaviors. This includes providing personal protective equipment, safety training materials, ergonomic tools, and access to safety professionals for guidance and assistance. By providing adequate resources and support, individuals feel empowered to prioritize safety and make informed decisions to protect themselves and their colleagues.

In summary, empowering individuals to take ownership of their attitudes towards safety involves providing education, fostering open communication, promoting leadership support, delegating responsibility, and providing resources and support. By empowering individuals at all levels of the organization, organizations can drive positive change, enhance safety culture, and create safer and healthier work environments for everyone.

SUMMARY OF CHAPTER 1: UNDERSTANDING ATTITUDE-BASED SAFETY

Chapter 1: Understanding Attitude-Based Safety delves into the foundational aspects of how attitudes influence safety behaviors and the overall safety culture within an organization.

1.1 The Power of Attitude in Safety

Attitudes wield significant influence over safety outcomes, as evidenced by real-life examples where positive attitudes have led to safer work environments and reduced accidents. By understanding the psychological mechanisms that underpin attitudes, including cognitive and emotional processes, organizations can leverage attitudes for change and drive meaningful improvements in safety.

1.2 Attitude Formation and Maintenance

Attitudes towards safety are shaped by a variety of factors, including past experiences, social influences, and organizational culture. By tracing the origins of attitudes, organizations can gain insights into how to nurture positive attitudes over time through ongoing education, communication, and reinforcement. Additionally, addressing negativity towards safety requires techniques such as open dialogue, empathy, and support to foster a culture of positivity and resilience.

1.3 Attitude as the Core Factor

Attitudes serve as the core factor driving effective safety practices and initiatives within organizations. By integrating attitudes into safety practices, organizations can establish a strong foundation for safety culture and align organizational values and objectives with a commitment to fostering positive safety attitudes. Empowering individuals at all levels of the organization to take ownership of their attitudes towards safety is crucial for driving positive change and creating a culture of safety where safety is prioritized and valued by everyone.

In summary, Chapter 1 emphasizes the importance of understanding, nurturing, and empowering attitudes towards safety to drive meaningful improvements in safety outcomes and create safer and healthier work environments for all individuals involved.

As we conclude Chapter 1, "Understanding Attitude-Based Safety," we recognize the pivotal role that attitudes play in shaping our safety behaviors. By examining the psychological mechanisms behind attitudes and their impact on workplace safety, we've gained a comprehensive understanding of how positive attitudes can significantly reduce accidents and foster a safer environment. We've also explored the origins of these attitudes, considering how past experiences, social influences, and organizational culture contribute to their formation. This foundational knowledge sets the stage for leveraging attitudes to drive safety improvements and integrate them into effective safety practices.

Transitioning into Chapter 2, "Developing Positive Safety Attitudes," we shift our focus from understanding the theoretical underpinnings of attitudes to actively cultivating them in our daily routines. Promoting safety awareness becomes crucial as we explore methods to create a culture of awareness through training, communication, and technology. By engaging the workforce and establishing clear expectations for safety responsibilities, we aim to build a robust culture of responsibility and mutual support. This chapter also emphasizes the critical influence of leadership in modeling and fostering positive safety attitudes, empowering leaders to drive safety initiatives and continuously improve safety practices across the organization.

Chapter 2: Developing Positive Safety Attitudes

Positive anything is better than negative nothing

- Elbert Hubbard

2.1 PROMOTING SAFETY AWARENESS

Promoting safety awareness is a foundational strategy in developing positive safety attitudes within an organization. By making employees conscious of safety risks and encouraging a culture of vigilance, organizations can cultivate attitudes that prioritize safety.

This section explores the methods and benefits of promoting safety awareness to develop positive safety attitudes.

2.1.1 Creating a Culture of Awareness: Explore methods for raising awareness of safety risks and hazards through training, communication, and visual reminders.

Raising awareness of safety risks and hazards is a fundamental step in developing positive safety attitudes within an organization. Awareness can be significantly enhanced through a combination of training, communication, and visual reminders.

Each method plays a unique role in ensuring that safety remains at the forefront of employees' minds, fostering a culture where safety is a shared value and priority.

Creating a culture of awareness involves instilling a proactive mindset towards safety across all levels of the organization can be achieved through various ways.

Training

Regular and comprehensive training sessions that cover various aspects of workplace safety as well as utilizing interactive methods like workshops, simulations, and e-learning modules to engage employees.

Comprehensive Safety Training Programs:

Implementing regular and comprehensive safety training programs is essential. These programs should cover general safety practices as well as job-specific hazards and procedures. Training sessions can be conducted through various formats such as workshops, seminars, online courses, and hands-on demonstrations. The goal is to equip employees with the knowledge and skills they need to identify and mitigate risks effectively.

Induction Training:

New employees should undergo thorough induction training that emphasizes the organization's commitment to safety. This training should introduce them to the company's safety policies, procedures, and the importance of maintaining a safe working environment from day one.

Ongoing Education:

Safety training should not be a one-time event. Regular refresher courses and updates are necessary to keep employees informed about new hazards, changes in procedures, and advancements in safety technology. Ongoing education reinforces the importance of safety and ensures that employees' knowledge remains current.

Scenario-Based Training:

Incorporating scenario-based training exercises can help employees practice their response to potential safety incidents. These exercises simulate real-life situations, allowing employees to develop their problem-solving skills and preparedness in a controlled environment.

Communication

Clear, consistent communication about safety policies, procedures, and expectations.

Utilizing multiple channels such as emails, newsletters, and intranet portals to disseminate safety information.

Open and Transparent Communication:

Effective communication is crucial in raising safety awareness. Organizations should foster an environment where open and transparent communication about safety is encouraged. This includes regular safety meetings, briefings, and discussions where employees can voice their concerns and share ideas.

Safety Bulletins and Newsletters:

Distributing safety bulletins and newsletters can keep safety at the forefront of employees' minds. These communications should include updates on safety policies, tips for safe practices, incident reports, and success stories of how safety measures have prevented accidents.

Safety Alerts and Notifications:

Utilize safety alerts and notifications to promptly inform employees about new hazards, procedural changes, or important safety reminders. These can be distributed through email, SMS, or internal communication platforms.

Feedback Mechanisms:

Establishing mechanisms for feedback allows employees to report safety concerns and suggest improvements. Anonymous feedback options can encourage more open reporting of potential issues without fear of retribution.

Visual Reminders

Visual Reminders:

Implementing posters, signs, and digital displays throughout the workplace to serve as constant safety reminders.

Using visuals that are easy to understand and capture attention effectively.

Safety Signage:

Strategically placed safety signs and posters around the workplace serve as constant visual reminders of the importance of safety. These signs should highlight key safety practices, emergency procedures, and hazard warnings.

Visual Management Tools:

Tools such as color-coded floor markings, labels, and safety boards can visually organize information and indicate safe pathways, hazardous zones, and equipment usage instructions. These tools help in creating an intuitive understanding of safety protocols.

Digital Displays:

Utilize digital displays and monitors to broadcast safety messages, reminders, and real-time safety data. These displays can show rotating safety tips, current safety metrics, and updates on safety initiatives, keeping the information fresh and engaging.

Infographics and Visual Aids:

Infographics and other visual aids can simplify complex safety information and make it more accessible. Use these tools to illustrate safety procedures, emergency response steps, and the proper use of personal protective equipment (PPE).

2.1.2 Engaging the Workforce: Discuss the importance of involving employees in safety initiatives and empowering them to actively contribute to safety awareness efforts.

Involving employees in safety initiatives is crucial for creating a culture of safety where everyone feels invested in maintaining a secure work environment. Empowering employees to actively contribute to safety awareness efforts can lead to increased engagement, improved morale, and ultimately, a safer workplace.

Why engaging the workforce is essential and how organizations can empower their employees for safety, is explained hereunder:

Importance of Employee Involvement

Ownership and Accountability:

When employees are actively involved in safety initiatives, they take ownership of their own safety and that of their colleagues. This sense of accountability fosters a culture where safety is everyone's responsibility.

Unique Insights and Perspectives:

Employees are often the ones performing the tasks on the front lines, making them valuable sources of insight into potential hazards and safety improvements. By encouraging their participation, organizations can tap into their knowledge and experience to identify risks and develop effective solutions.

Increased Awareness and Compliance:

Engaging employees in safety initiatives raises awareness about safety practices and procedures, leading to higher compliance rates. When employees understand the reasons behind safety measures and feel involved in the decision-making process, they are more likely to adhere to safety protocols.

Strategies for Empowering Employees

Participation in Safety Committee Meetings:

Encourage employees to participate in safety committee meetings where they can discuss safety issues, brainstorm solutions, and provide feedback on safety policies and procedures. These meetings should be inclusive and provide opportunities for all employees to contribute their ideas.

Open Channels for Communication:

Create open channels for communication where employees can freely share their opinions, concerns, and suggestions related to safety. This can include suggestion boxes, anonymous reporting systems, or regular safety forums where employees can voice their thoughts.

Recognition and Rewards:

Recognize and reward employees for their contributions to safety awareness efforts. This can take the form of verbal praise, certificates of appreciation, or even "best idea" awards for innovative safety suggestions. Recognizing employees' efforts reinforces the importance of safety and encourages continued engagement.

Training and Education:

Provide employees with training and education opportunities to enhance their knowledge of safety practices and procedures. This can include workshops, seminars, or online courses on topics such as hazard identification, emergency response, and risk management.

Promote Peer-to-Peer Support:

Encourage peer-to-peer support by fostering a culture where employees feel comfortable looking out for each other's safety. Encourage team members to remind each other of safety procedures and intervene if they observe unsafe behaviors.

Benefits of Empowering Employees

Improved Safety Culture:

Empowering employees for safety creates a culture where safety is valued and prioritized by everyone in the organization. This leads to fewer accidents, lower injury rates, and a safer work environment overall.

Increased Morale and Job Satisfaction:

When employees feel empowered to contribute to safety initiatives, it boosts their morale and job satisfaction. They feel more engaged in their work and proud to be part of an organization that values their input.

Enhanced Problem-Solving Capabilities:

Involving employees in safety initiatives enhances their problem-solving capabilities as they collaborate to identify and address safety issues. This fosters a culture of continuous improvement where safety processes are regularly evaluated and refined.

Engaging the workforce and empowering employees for safety is essential for creating a culture of safety where everyone plays an active role in maintaining a secure work environment.

By involving employees in safety initiatives, organizations can leverage their unique insights and perspectives, increase awareness and compliance, and ultimately, achieve better safety outcomes for all.

By encouraging participation in safety committee meetings, providing open channels for communication, recognizing employees' contributions, offering training and education opportunities, and promoting peer-to-peer support, organizations can empower their employees to be active participants in safety awareness efforts, leading to a safer and healthier workplace for everyone.

2.1.3 Leveraging Technology: Highlight the role of technology in promoting safety awareness, such as mobile apps, virtual reality simulations, and data analytics.

Technology can significantly enhance safety awareness by providing innovative tools and resources, like:

Mobile Apps:

Virtual Reality (VR) Simulations:

Data Analytics:

In today's digital age, technology plays a pivotal role in promoting safety awareness and enhancing workplace safety. By harnessing the power of innovative tools and platforms, organizations can effectively communicate safety information, simulate hazardous scenarios, and analyze safety data to identify risks and prevent accidents.

Here's how technology is revolutionizing safety awareness:

Mobile Apps for On-the-Go Safety

Accessibility and Convenience:

Mobile apps provide instant access to safety information, allowing employees to review procedures, report hazards, and receive real-time alerts regardless of their location. This accessibility ensures that safety resources are readily available whenever and wherever they are needed.

Interactive Training Modules:

Many mobile apps offer interactive training modules that engage users with multimedia content, quizzes, and simulations.

These immersive learning experiences enhance retention and comprehension of safety concepts, making training more effective and engaging for employees.

Communication and Collaboration:

Mobile apps facilitate communication and collaboration among employees, enabling them to share safety tips, report incidents, and communicate with safety personnel in real time. This instant connectivity fosters a culture of safety where information is readily exchanged, and potential hazards are quickly addressed.

Virtual Reality Simulations for Immersive Training

Realistic Hazard Scenarios:

Virtual reality (VR) simulations immerse users in realistic hazard scenarios, allowing them to experience potential dangers firsthand in a safe and controlled environment. By simulating hazardous situations, VR training prepares employees to recognize and respond to risks effectively.

Hands-On Learning:

VR simulations offer a hands-on learning experience where users can practice safety procedures, such as emergency evacuations or equipment operation, in a virtual setting. This hands-on approach enhances muscle memory and decision-making skills, improving readiness for real-world emergencies.

Behavioral Analysis and Feedback:

VR simulations can track user behavior and provide immediate feedback on performance, allowing trainers to assess competency and identify areas for improvement. This data-driven approach enables targeted training interventions and ensures that employees are adequately prepared to mitigate safety risks.

Data Analytics for Predictive Insights

Risk Identification and Assessment:

Data analytics tools analyze vast amounts of safety data, including incident reports, near misses, and safety observations, to identify trends and patterns indicative of potential risks. By proactively identifying hazards, organizations can implement preventive measures to mitigate the likelihood of accidents.

Predictive Modeling:

Advanced analytics techniques, such as predictive modeling and machine learning, forecast future safety outcomes based on historical data and risk factors. These predictive insights enable organizations to anticipate safety challenges and allocate resources more effectively to prevent accidents before they occur.

Continuous Improvement:

Data analytics facilitate continuous improvement by providing actionable insights for optimizing safety processes and procedures. By monitoring key performance indicators and benchmarking against industry standards, organizations can iteratively refine their safety programs to achieve better outcomes over time.

By leveraging technology, organizations can revolutionize safety awareness and empower employees to make informed decisions that protect their well-being in the workplace.

Whether through mobile apps for on-the-go safety, virtual reality simulations for immersive training, or data analytics for predictive insights, technology offers a wealth of opportunities to enhance safety awareness and prevent accidents.

By embracing these innovative tools and platforms, organizations can create safer and healthier work environments for all.

2.2 Building a Culture of Responsibility

Employer's Responsibility: Creating an Environment of Safety

Leadership Commitment:

In any organization, the tone for safety culture is set at the top. Leaders must exhibit an unwavering commitment to safety, which should be evident in their daily actions and decisions. This commitment is not only about setting policies but also about embodying the principles of safety through consistent behavior.

Leaders must actively participate in safety programs, communicate the importance of safety in every interaction, and ensure that safety is integrated into all organizational processes.

Policy and Procedure Development:

Employers must develop comprehensive safety policies and procedures that are clear, accessible, and enforceable. These policies should be formulated with input from all levels of the organization to ensure they are practical and effective. Regular reviews and updates of these policies are essential to adapt to new challenges and innovations in safety practices.

Resource Allocation:

Adequate resources must be allocated to safety initiatives. This includes investing in safety training programs, safety equipment, and technology that enhances safety monitoring and reporting.

Employers should ensure that financial and human resources dedicated to safety are sufficient to maintain high standards.

Empowering Safety Leaders:

Designating safety leaders or champions within the organization can reinforce the commitment to safety. These individuals should be empowered with the authority and resources to lead safety initiatives, conduct training, and monitor compliance.

They act as the bridge between management and employees, ensuring that safety remains a priority.

Employees' Responsibility: Ownership and Engagement

Active Participation:

Employees must take an active role in their safety and the safety of their colleagues. This involves participating in safety training, adhering to safety protocols, and being vigilant about potential hazards.

Employees should feel empowered to speak up about safety concerns and suggest improvements without fear of retribution.

Peer Support and Accountability:

A culture of responsibility thrives when employees support and hold each other accountable. Peer-to-peer interactions are crucial in reinforcing safe behaviors and attitudes. Encouraging open dialogue about safety among employees can lead to a more cohesive and proactive safety culture.

Continuous Learning:

Safety is an ongoing learning process. Employees should be encouraged to continuously update their knowledge and skills related to safety.

This can be achieved through regular training sessions, safety drills, and staying informed about the latest safety practices and technologies.

Personal Responsibility: Individual Commitment to Safety

Self-Reflection:

Individuals must engage in self-reflection to understand their attitudes towards safety. This involves assessing one's own behaviors, recognizing areas for improvement, and committing to personal growth in safety practices. Personal responsibility starts with acknowledging that safety is not just an organizational mandate but a personal commitment.

Adopting Safe Practices:

Incorporating safe practices into daily routines is essential. This includes wearing appropriate safety gear, following established safety procedures, and being mindful of one's actions and their impact on the safety of others. Personal responsibility means consistently choosing to act in a manner that prioritizes safety, even when it might be inconvenient.

Encouraging a Positive Attitude:

Attitude plays a crucial role in safety. A positive attitude towards safety can significantly influence one's behavior and the behavior of others. Individuals should strive to maintain a proactive and positive attitude towards safety, encouraging their peers to do the same.

Key Takeaways in building a culture of responsibility.

Leadership Commitment: Leaders set the tone for safety by embodying and enforcing safety principles.

Policy Development: Comprehensive and practical safety policies are essential for guiding organizational safety practices.

Resource Allocation: Adequate resources must be dedicated to safety initiatives to maintain high standards.

Active Participation: Employees play a crucial role in their safety and should actively engage in safety practices and initiatives.

Self-Reflection and Personal Commitment: Personal responsibility starts with self-reflection and committing to adopting safe practices and a positive attitude towards safety.

Action Steps

For Employers:

Demonstrate commitment to safety through actions and decisions.

Develop and regularly update comprehensive safety policies.

Allocate sufficient resources to safety initiatives.

Empower safety leaders within the organization.

For Employees:

Actively participate in safety training and initiatives.

Support and hold peers accountable for safety.

Engage in continuous learning about safety practices.

For Individuals:

Reflect on personal attitudes and behaviors towards safety.

Consistently adopt and practice safe behaviors.

Maintain a positive attitude towards safety and encourage others to do the same.

By fostering a culture of responsibility at every level, organizations can create a safer and more productive work environment. This shared commitment to safety ensures that everyone plays a role in maintaining and enhancing safety standards.

2.2.1 Establishing Clear Expectations: Outline the importance of setting clear expectations for safety responsibilities and accountability at all levels of the organization.

Setting clear expectations for safety responsibilities and accountability is paramount to building a culture of responsibility within an organization. Here's why:

Clarity and Consistency: Clear expectations ensure that all employees understand their roles and responsibilities regarding safety. By outlining specific tasks, procedures, and standards, organizations provide clarity on what is expected of each individual, fostering consistency in safety practices.

Accountability and Ownership: When expectations are clearly defined, employees are more likely to take ownership of their safety responsibilities. Clear guidelines establish accountability for safety performance, encouraging individuals to proactively identify hazards, adhere to procedures, and intervene in unsafe situations.

Alignment with Organizational Goals: Setting clear expectations aligns safety initiatives with broader organizational goals and objectives. By emphasizing the importance of safety as a core value, organizations demonstrate their commitment to protecting the well-being of their employees and achieving excellence in safety performance.

Promotion of Positive Behavior: Clear expectations serve as a catalyst for promoting positive safety behavior throughout the organization. When employees understand the standards for safe conduct, they are more inclined to adhere to guidelines, follow procedures, and actively contribute to a culture of responsibility.

Prevention of Misunderstandings and Conflicts: Ambiguity regarding safety responsibilities can lead to misunderstandings, conflicts, and ultimately, safety incidents. By clearly articulating expectations, organizations minimize the risk of misinterpretation and ensure that everyone is on the same page when it comes to safety protocols.

In summary, establishing clear expectations for safety responsibility is essential for creating a culture of accountability, ownership, and proactive safety behavior within an organization. By clearly defining roles, setting standards, and aligning safety initiatives with organizational goals, organizations can foster a culture where safety is everyone's responsibility, leading to safer work environments and improved overall performance.

2.2.2 Encouraging Peer Support: Discuss the value of peer-to-peer support and accountability in fostering a culture of responsibility and mutual safety.

Peer support plays a crucial role in fostering a culture of responsibility and mutual safety within an organization. Here's why encouraging peer support is essential:

Shared Responsibility: Peer support reinforces the idea that safety is everyone's responsibility. When employees actively support and look out for each other, they create a collective sense of ownership over safety, leading to a more proactive approach to hazard identification and risk mitigation.

Social Norms and Influence: Humans are highly influenced by their peers and social circles. Encouraging peer support for safety behaviors can help establish positive safety norms within the workplace. When employees observe their colleague's prioritizing safety and supporting one another, they are more likely to emulate those behaviors, creating a ripple effect throughout the organization.

Increased Awareness and Vigilance: Peer support enhances safety awareness and vigilance by encouraging employees to actively engage in safety-related discussions and observations.

When colleagues collaborate to identify potential hazards and share best practices, they contribute to a more robust safety culture where everyone is alert and proactive in preventing accidents.

Emotional Support and Encouragement: Peer support provides emotional support and encouragement during challenging or high-risk situations. Knowing that they have the backing of their peers can empower employees to speak up about safety concerns, seek assistance when needed, and take decisive action to prevent accidents or injuries.

Accountability and Feedback: Peer support fosters a culture of accountability by holding individuals accountable for their safety behaviors.

When employees hold each other accountable and provide constructive feedback, they create a culture where safety is non-negotiable, and everyone is committed to upholding high standards of safety performance.

In summary, encouraging peer support for safety is instrumental in creating a culture of responsibility, collaboration, and mutual support within an organization. By leveraging the influence of peers, organizations can promote positive safety behaviors, increase awareness, and ultimately, enhance safety outcomes for all employees.

2.2.3 Recognizing and Rewarding Responsibility: Provide examples of effective recognition and reward systems that reinforce positive safety attitudes and behaviors.

Recognizing and rewarding responsibility is a powerful way to reinforce positive safety attitudes and behaviors within an organization. Here are examples of effective recognition and reward systems:

Safety Achievement Awards: Implement an awards program that recognizes individuals or teams for outstanding safety achievements. Awards could include "Safety Star of the Month" or "Safety Champion of the Year," accompanied by tangible rewards such as gift cards, certificates, or plaques.

Safety Bonuses or Incentives: Offer monetary bonuses or incentives to employees who consistently demonstrate exemplary safety behaviors. This could involve rewarding individuals or departments that achieve specific safety milestones, such as a certain number of days without accidents or near misses.

Peer Recognition Programs: Establish a peer-to-peer recognition program where employees can nominate their colleagues for demonstrating exceptional safety practices. Peer nominations provide valuable feedback and encouragement, fostering a culture of mutual recognition and support.

Safety Points System: Implement a points-based system where employees earn points for actively participating in safety activities, attending training sessions, reporting hazards, or suggesting safety improvements. Accumulated points can be redeemed for rewards or privileges within the organization.

Safety Excellence Certifications: Offer formal certifications or badges to employees who undergo specialized safety training, demonstrate mastery of safety procedures, or consistently adhere to safety protocols. These certifications serve as tangible evidence of individual commitment to safety excellence.

Public Recognition and Celebrations: Recognize safety achievements publicly through company-wide meetings, newsletters, or social media platforms. Celebrate milestones such as reaching a significant number of accident-free days or successfully implementing a new safety initiative.

Safety Leadership Awards: Acknowledge and reward supervisors, managers, or safety leaders who actively promote and support a culture of safety within their teams. Leadership recognition reinforces the importance of top-down commitment to safety and encourages managerial involvement in safety initiatives.

Team-Based Rewards: Encourage teamwork and collaboration by offering rewards for collective safety achievements. Recognize entire departments or work units that demonstrate exceptional safety performance or collaborate effectively to address safety challenges.

Continuous Improvement Recognition: Emphasize the importance of continuous improvement by rewarding individuals or teams that identify safety hazards, propose innovative solutions, or contribute to ongoing safety initiatives.

Personalized Rewards: Tailor rewards individual preferences or interests to increase their significance and motivational impact. Consider offering a range of rewards options, allowing employees to choose rewards that are meaningful to them.

By implementing effective recognition and reward systems, organizations can reinforce positive safety attitudes and behaviors, cultivate a culture of responsibility, and ultimately, improve overall safety performance and outcomes.

Safety Excellence Luncheons: Host periodic luncheons or banquets to honor individuals or teams who have made significant contributions to safety. These events provide an opportunity for senior leaders to personally thank employees for their dedication to safety and publicly recognize their achievements.

Safety Wall of Fame: Establish a "Wall of Fame" or bulletin board prominently displayed in the workplace, featuring photographs and profiles of employees who have demonstrated exemplary safety practices. This visual display serves as a constant reminder of the organization's commitment to safety and celebrates the individuals who embody this commitment.

Safety Hero Spotlight: Shine a spotlight on safety heroes by featuring their stories in company newsletters, intranet articles, or social media posts. Highlight their proactive safety initiatives, quick thinking in emergency situations, or innovative solutions to safety challenges to inspire others and reinforce desired behaviors.

Safety Training Scholarships: Offer scholarships or financial assistance for employees to pursue advanced safety training, certifications, or professional development opportunities. Investing in employees' ongoing education and skill development demonstrates the organization's commitment to safety excellence and empowers individuals to enhance their safety knowledge and expertise.

Safety Ambassador Program: Establish a Safety Ambassador Program where select employees serve as safety ambassadors or mentors to their peers. These ambassadors receive specialized training and resources to promote safety awareness, provide guidance on safety best practices, and serve as role models for their colleagues.

Safety Performance Contests: Organize friendly competitions or challenges focused on safety performance metrics, such as the most creative hazard identification, the highest participation in safety training, or the most effective implementation of safety procedures. Encourage healthy competition among teams or departments to achieve safety goals and foster a sense of camaraderie.

Personalized Safety Gear: Provide personalized safety gear or equipment upgrades as rewards for exceptional safety performance. Engraved or customized safety helmets, gloves, or protective eyewear not only enhance safety but also serve as tangible symbols of recognition and appreciation.

Safety Achievement Badges: Introduce a badge or pin system where employees earn badges for achieving specific safety milestones or completing safety-related tasks. Employees can proudly display these badges on their uniforms or work attire, symbolizing their commitment to safety excellence.

Safety Family Day: Organize a special event, such as a Safety Family Day or picnic, where employees and their families can come together to celebrate safety achievements and learn about safety practices in a fun and interactive environment. Incorporate games, activities, and demonstrations to engage both adults and children in safety awareness.

Safety Book Club: Launch a Safety Book Club where employees read and discuss books, articles, or case studies related to safety culture, leadership, or best practices. Encourage dialogue and reflection on key safety concepts, and reward participants with book-themed prizes or certificates of participation.

By implementing a variety of recognition and reward initiatives tailored to the organization's culture and objectives, leaders can foster a positive safety culture, motivate employees to prioritize safety, and drive continuous improvement in safety performance.

2.3.1 Leading by Example: Emphasize the critical role of leadership in modeling positive safety attitudes and behaviors for the rest of the organization.

Leading by example is one of the most powerful ways for leaders to influence attitudes and behaviors within an organization. Here's how leaders can effectively demonstrate positive safety attitudes and behaviors:

Active Participation: Leaders should actively participate in safety initiatives and programs to demonstrate their commitment to safety. This could involve regularly joining safety observation programs on the work floor, actively engaging in safety committee meetings, and participating in safety training sessions alongside employees.

Open Communication: Leaders should foster an environment of open communication where safety concerns can be freely discussed and addressed. By encouraging employees to voice their opinions and ideas regarding safety issues, leaders demonstrate their willingness to listen and collaborate on finding solutions.

Accessibility: Leaders should make themselves accessible to employees to discuss safety matters and address any concerns that may arise. This accessibility can help employees feel valued and supported in their safety efforts, fostering a sense of trust and collaboration within the organization.

Visibility: Leaders should make their commitment to safety visible throughout the organization. This could involve visibly displaying safety messages and reminders, wearing appropriate personal protective equipment (PPE) when required, and actively participating in safety inspections and audits.

Consistency: Consistency is key to effective leadership. Leaders should consistently prioritize safety in their decision-making processes, actions, and communications. By consistently demonstrating a commitment to safety, leaders set a positive example for employees to follow.

Recognition: Leaders should recognize and reward employees for their safety contributions and achievements. By publicly acknowledging and celebrating individuals and teams who demonstrate positive safety attitudes and behaviors, leaders reinforce the importance of safety within the organization.

Continuous Improvement: Leaders should actively seek opportunities for continuous improvement in safety practices and processes. This could involve soliciting feedback from employees, conducting regular safety assessments, and investing in resources and training to support ongoing safety initiatives.

Empowerment: Leaders should empower employees to take ownership of safety by involving them in decision-making processes and encouraging them to identify and address safety hazards proactively. Empowered employees are more likely to demonstrate positive safety attitudes and behaviors, knowing that their input is valued, and their actions contribute to a safer work environment.

Training and Development: Leaders should invest in training and development programs that equip employees with the knowledge, skills, and resources needed to prioritize safety in their daily tasks.

By providing comprehensive safety training, leaders demonstrate their commitment to employee well-being and equip individuals with the tools they need to adopt and maintain positive safety attitudes.

Continuous Communication: Effective communication is essential for fostering positive safety attitudes within an organization. Leaders should communicate safety expectations clearly and regularly, providing updates on safety initiatives, sharing relevant information about safety hazards and risks, and reinforcing the importance of safety in all aspects of the work environment.

By maintaining open and transparent communication channels, leaders can ensure that safety remains a top priority for everyone in the organization.

By leading by example and emphasizing the importance of positive safety attitudes and behaviors, leaders can create a culture of safety where every individual feels empowered to prioritize safety in their daily actions and decisions.

2.3.2 Empowering Leaders: Discuss strategies for empowering leaders to effectively communicate safety expectations, provide support, and promote a culture of safety.

Empowering leaders to promote a culture of safety involves providing them with the tools, resources, and support needed to effectively lead safety initiatives within their teams. Here are some strategies for empowering leaders:

Training and Education: Offer comprehensive training and education programs to equip leaders with the knowledge and skills necessary to champion safety in the workplace. This training should cover topics such as hazard recognition, risk assessment, safety regulations, and effective communication techniques.

Clear Expectations: Clearly define the role of leaders in promoting safety and communicate clear expectations for their responsibilities in this area. Leaders should understand that safety is a priority and that they play a crucial role in fostering a culture of safety within their teams.

Supportive Environment: Create a supportive environment where leaders feel comfortable discussing safety concerns, addressing issues, and seeking assistance when needed. Encourage open communication and provide avenues for leaders to voice their opinions, share best practices, and collaborate with their peers.

Resources and Tools: Provide leaders with access to resources and tools that facilitate safety management and decision-making. This may include safety manuals, procedures, checklists, incident reporting systems, and access to safety experts or consultants.

Recognition and Incentives: Recognize and reward leaders who demonstrate a commitment to safety and actively promote a culture of safety within their teams. This could involve acknowledging their contributions in team meetings, providing public recognition, or offering incentives for achieving safety goals.

Continual Improvement: Encourage leaders to continually evaluate and improve their safety leadership skills through feedback, self-assessment, and professional development opportunities. Foster a culture of learning and growth where leaders are encouraged to seek out new knowledge and best practices in safety management.

By empowering leaders with the necessary training, support, resources, and recognition, organizations can cultivate a cadre of safety-conscious leaders who are capable of driving positive change and fostering a safer work environment for all employees.

2.3.3 Training and Development: Highlight the importance of leadership training and development programs that emphasize safety leadership skills and behaviors.

Training and development programs for leaders play a crucial role in emphasizing safety leadership skills and behaviors. Here's how:

Skill Enhancement: Leadership training programs focus on enhancing specific safety leadership skills and behaviors, such as effective communication, conflict resolution, decision-making, and problem-solving. These skills are essential for leaders to effectively manage safety initiatives and address safety-related issues within their teams.

Understanding Safety Regulations: Training programs provide leaders with a thorough understanding of safety regulations, standards, and best practices relevant to their industry. This knowledge enables leaders to ensure compliance with safety requirements and proactively identify and mitigate safety risks in the workplace.

Risk Management: Leaders learn how to assess and manage safety risks effectively through training programs. They gain the necessary tools and techniques to identify hazards, conduct risk assessments, and implement control measures to prevent accidents and injuries.

Creating a Safety Culture: Training programs emphasize the importance of fostering a strong safety culture within the organization. Leaders learn how to promote safety awareness, encourage employee engagement, and cultivate a supportive environment where safety is prioritized and valued by all.

Leading by Example: Leadership training emphasizes the importance of leading by example when it comes to safety. Leaders are encouraged to demonstrate safe behaviors, follow safety protocols, and actively participate in safety initiatives to set a positive example for their team members.

Continuous Improvement: Training and development programs promote a culture of continuous improvement by providing leaders with opportunities to reflect on their safety leadership practices, receive feedback, and identify areas for growth. Leaders are encouraged to seek out ongoing learning opportunities and stay updated on emerging trends and best practices in safety leadership.

By investing in comprehensive training and development programs for leaders, organizations can equip them with the knowledge, skills, and mindset needed to effectively lead safety initiatives and create a safer work environment for everyone.

SUMMARY OF CHAPTER 2: DEVELOPING POSITIVE SAFETY ATTITUDES

In Chapter 2, we explore strategies for fostering positive safety attitudes within organizations, focusing on promoting safety awareness, building a culture of responsibility, and harnessing leadership's influence on attitudes.

2.1 Promoting Safety Awareness

Safety awareness is the foundation of a strong safety culture. We explore various methods for raising awareness of safety risks and hazards, including comprehensive training programs, effective communication strategies, and the use of visual reminders such as signage and posters. By creating a culture of awareness, organizations empower employees to recognize and mitigate safety hazards proactively.

2.2 Building a Culture of Responsibility

A culture of responsibility is essential for ensuring that every individual takes ownership of their safety and the safety of others. We discuss the importance of setting clear expectations for safety responsibilities and accountability at all levels of the organization. Additionally, we explore the value of peer-to-peer support and accountability in fostering a collective commitment to safety. Furthermore, we highlight the significance of recognizing and rewarding responsible behavior to reinforce positive safety attitudes.

2.3 Leadership's Influence on Attitudes

Leadership plays a crucial role in shaping organizational attitudes towards safety. We emphasize the importance of leaders leading by example, demonstrating a commitment to safety through their actions and decisions. Additionally, we provide strategies for empowering leaders to effectively communicate safety expectations, provide support, and promote a culture of safety within their teams. Furthermore, we highlight the role of leadership training and development programs in equipping leaders with the necessary skills and behaviors to drive positive safety attitudes throughout the organization.

In Chapter 2, readers will gain valuable insights into how to promote safety awareness, foster a culture of responsibility, and leverage leadership's influence to develop positive safety attitudes within their organizations. Through practical examples and actionable strategies, readers will be empowered to create safer work environments and cultivate a culture of safety excellence.

As we conclude our exploration of developing positive safety attitudes, it's clear that promoting safety awareness, building a culture of responsibility, and leveraging leadership's influence are foundational elements in creating a robust safety culture. By utilizing various methods to raise awareness of safety risks and hazards, engaging the workforce in safety initiatives, and employing cutting-edge technology, organizations can significantly enhance their safety practices.

Furthermore, establishing clear expectations, encouraging peer support, and recognizing responsible behaviors play a crucial role in fostering a culture of responsibility and mutual safety. Leadership's proactive involvement in modeling, empowering, and training further solidifies the commitment to safety throughout the organization.

However, even with these positive measures in place, challenges remain. In the next chapter, we will delve into overcoming the barriers that can hinder the adoption and maintenance of positive safety attitudes. Understanding resistance to change, addressing negative attitudes, and fostering resilience are essential steps in ensuring that the safety culture continues to evolve and improve.

By addressing these barriers head-on and providing practical strategies for change, organizations can pave the way for a safer, more supportive work environment. Let's now transition to Chapter 3: Overcoming Attitude Barriers, where we will explore these critical aspects in detail and provide actionable insights for navigating and mitigating resistance to safety initiatives.

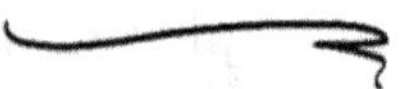

Chapter 3: Overcoming Attitude Barriers

Strength and growth come only through continuous effort and struggle

- Napoleon Hill

Understanding Attitude Barriers

In this chapter we focus on various barriers that can obstruct the development and maintenance of positive safety attitudes. These barriers can stem from individual psychological factors, organizational culture, or external influences.

Some key attitude barriers are as follows:

1. Resistance to Change

Fear of the Unknown: Individuals may resist safety initiatives due to fear of unfamiliar processes or outcomes. This fear can stem from a lack of understanding or previous negative experiences with change.

Loss of Control: When safety measures are implemented, employees might feel they are losing control over their work environment or methods, leading to resistance.

Perceived Inconvenience: Some safety protocols might be seen as cumbersome or time-consuming, leading employees to resist them in favor of more familiar, albeit less safe, practices.

2. Negative Attitudes

Complacency: Over time, employees might become complacent, believing that accidents won't happen to them because they haven't experienced any serious incidents.

Cynicism: Past experiences with ineffective safety programs or management's inconsistent commitment to safety can breed cynicism among employees, leading them to doubt the efficacy of new initiatives.

Peer Pressure: Workers might face pressure from colleagues to conform to unsafe behaviors, especially if such behaviors are normalized within the group.

3. Organizational Culture

Lack of Support from Management: If the leadership does not actively support and prioritize safety, employees are likely to follow suit, viewing safety measures as unimportant.

Inadequate Training and Resources: Without proper training and resources, employees may feel ill-equipped to follow safety protocols, leading to frustration and non-compliance.

Inconsistent Enforcement: Inconsistent application of safety rules can create confusion and resentment, undermining the overall safety culture.

4. External Influences

Economic Pressure: Financial constraints or production pressures can lead to shortcuts and unsafe practices, as the focus shifts to output rather than safety.

Regulatory Changes: Constant changes in safety regulations can overwhelm employees, leading to confusion and resistance to adopting new practices.

Overcoming Attitude Barriers

Addressing these barriers requires a multifaceted approach that includes effective communication, empathy, and support. In the following sections of Chapter 3, we will explore strategies to mitigate these barriers and foster a culture where positive safety attitudes can thrive. By understanding and tackling these barriers, organizations can create an environment where safety is not just a priority, but a fundamental value shared by all.

Internal and External Barriers to Positive Attitude:

To cultivate a positive safety attitude within an organization, it is crucial to understand and address both internal and external barriers. These barriers can impede the development and maintenance of a safety-first mindset. Here is a detailed exploration of each:

Internal Barriers

Internal barriers are obstacles that arise from within the individual or the organization. They are often psychological or cultural in nature and can significantly impact an employee's attitude towards safety.

Psychological Factors:

Fear of Change: Employees may be afraid of new safety protocols or changes in procedures, fearing they will make mistakes or face additional challenges.

Complacency: Individuals may develop a false sense of security, thinking that because accidents haven't happened to them in the past, they won't happen in the future.

Cynicism: Past experiences with ineffective safety measures can lead to a lack of trust in new safety initiatives, fostering a cynical attitude towards them.

Resistance to Authority: Some employees may resist safety directives simply because they come from management, viewing them as unnecessary impositions.

Cultural Factors:

Normalization of Deviance: Over time, deviations from safety protocols may become normalized, leading employees to view unsafe practices as acceptable.

Peer Pressure: Employees might feel pressured by colleagues to conform to unsafe behaviors to fit in or avoid conflict.

Inconsistent Messaging: Mixed messages from leadership regarding the importance of safety can create confusion and reduce the perceived importance of following safety protocols.

Organizational Factors:

Lack of Training: Inadequate training in safety procedures can leave employees feeling unprepared and insecure about implementing safety measures.

Inconsistent Enforcement: When safety rules are not consistently enforced, it undermines their importance and employees may not take them seriously.

Insufficient Resources: Lack of necessary safety equipment or resources can make it difficult for employees to adhere to safety protocols.

External Barriers

External barriers originate outside the individual or organization and can influence attitudes and behaviors related to safety.

Economic Pressures:

Cost-Cutting Measures: Financial constraints can lead to reduced spending on safety equipment, training, and personnel, increasing the risk of accidents.

Production Pressures: High demands for productivity can lead to shortcuts and neglect of safety protocols to meet deadlines.

Regulatory Environment:

Frequent Changes in Regulations: Constant updates to safety regulations can overwhelm employees and make it challenging to stay compliant.

Enforcement Variability: Inconsistent enforcement of safety regulations by external bodies can lead to uncertainty and inconsistent adherence to safety practices.

Industry Standards:

Competitive Pressure: In highly competitive industries, there may be pressure to cut corners to maintain an edge, compromising safety.

Benchmarking: If industry benchmarks do not prioritize safety, organizations might downplay the importance of robust safety practices.

Addressing Internal and External Barriers

Successfully overcoming these barriers involves a comprehensive approach that includes:

Effective Communication: Clearly communicating the importance of safety and the rationale behind safety protocols can help mitigate fear and resistance.

Training and Education: Providing thorough training and continuous education ensures that employees feel competent and confident in following safety procedures.

Leadership Commitment: Strong, visible commitment from leadership to prioritize and model safety can influence the entire organization's attitude towards safety.

Support Systems: Implementing support systems like peer support groups, counseling, and employee assistance programs can help address psychological barriers.

Resource Allocation: Ensuring that adequate resources are allocated for safety measures can address economic pressures and organizational resource gaps.

Consistent Enforcement and Adaptability: Regularly updating and consistently enforcing safety regulations and practices can help manage the external regulatory environment and industry standards.

By addressing these internal and external barriers, organizations can foster a culture where positive safety attitudes are developed and maintained, ultimately leading to a safer work environment.

3.1 Addressing Resistance to Change

3.1.1 Understanding Resistance: Explore common reasons for resistance to safety-related changes, such as fear of the unknown, loss of control, and perceived inconvenience.

Resistance to change is a common challenge when implementing safety-related changes within an organization. Understanding the underlying reasons for this resistance is the first step in addressing and overcoming it. Here are some common reasons for resistance to safety-related changes, along with examples and explanations:

1. Fear of the Unknown

Illustration: Imagine a factory that decides to implement a new safety protocol for operating machinery. Employees, used to the old way of doing things, may resist the new protocol simply because it is unfamiliar.

Explanation: The fear of the unknown is a natural human reaction to change. When employees are uncertain about what the new safety protocols entail or how they will affect their daily routines, they may become anxious and resistant. This fear can stem from concerns about their ability to adapt to new procedures, potential repercussions for non-compliance, or simply the discomfort of stepping out of their comfort zones.

Example: An assembly line worker might worry that new safety procedures will slow down production, impacting their performance metrics and potentially their job security.

2. Loss of Control

Illustration: In a construction company, management decides to enforce stricter safety measures, including mandatory safety checklists before using any heavy equipment. Some experienced workers resist, feeling that their autonomy and expertise are being undermined.

Explanation: Changes in safety protocols can make employees feel like they are losing control over their work environment. This is especially true if they perceive the changes as micromanagement or as a sign that their skills and judgment are not trusted. The sense of autonomy is important for job satisfaction and motivation, and any perceived threat to this autonomy can lead to resistance.

Example: A seasoned crane operator might feel that following a new, detailed safety checklist is unnecessary and a slight to their professional experience and judgment.

3. Perceived Inconvenience

Illustration: A hospital introduces a new set of hygiene protocols requiring additional handwashing and sanitizing steps. Nurses and doctors, already stretched thin by their workloads, see these new protocols as an added burden that takes time away from patient care.

Explanation: Employees might resist safety-related changes if they perceive them as inconvenient or add extra steps to their already busy schedules. If the new safety measures are seen as cumbersome or time-consuming, employees might push back, believing that these changes will hinder their efficiency and productivity.

Example: Medical staff might argue that the new hygiene protocols are impractical in emergency situations where every second counts.

4. Lack of Trust in Leadership

Illustration: Employees at a manufacturing plant might resist new safety protocols if they do not trust that the management has their best interests at heart.

Explanation: If there is a history of poor communication, broken promises, or perceived negligence by leadership, employees may be skeptical of any new initiatives, including those related to safety. Trust is a fundamental component of any successful change management process, and its absence can lead to significant resistance.

Example: Workers might believe that new safety measures are being implemented only to avoid regulatory fines, rather than to genuinely protect their well-being.

5. Past Negative Experiences

Illustration: A construction company that previously introduced a flawed safety protocol may find employees resistant to new changes due to memories of past failures.

Explanation: Negative experiences with previous safety changes can leave employees feeling cynical and doubtful about the effectiveness of new initiatives. If past changes were poorly implemented or resulted in negative outcomes, employees might be reluctant to embrace new efforts.

Example: Employees may remember a past initiative that led to confusion and inefficiency, leading them to distrust any new proposals.

6. Misunderstanding or Lack of Information

Illustration: In a healthcare setting, a new safety protocol might be resisted simply because staff do not fully understand how it works or why it is necessary.

Explanation: When employees are not given sufficient information about the nature and purpose of the changes, they are likely to resist out of confusion or ignorance. Clear, thorough communication is essential to ensure understanding and buy-in.

Example: A nurse might oppose a new sanitation procedure because they are unaware of the specific health benefits it provides.

7. Job Security Concerns

Illustration: In an industrial environment, workers might fear that new automated safety systems could eventually lead to job cuts.

Explanation: Changes that introduce new technology or alter existing workflows can create anxiety about job security. Employees might worry that the new safety measures are a step towards reducing the workforce or changing their roles in ways that they find undesirable.

Example: Machine operators might resist new automated safety systems, fearing that their roles will become obsolete.

8. Peer Pressure

Illustration: A new safety policy in a warehouse might be met with resistance if the dominant workplace culture is dismissive of safety rules.

Explanation: Peer pressure and the desire to conform to group norms can significantly influence individual behavior. If the prevailing attitude among colleagues is one of disregard for safety protocols, individuals might resist changes to avoid standing out or being ostracized.

Example: Workers might avoid wearing personal protective equipment because their peers consider it unnecessary or uncool.

9. Habit and Comfort with the Status Quo

Illustration: Office employees might resist a new ergonomic workstation setup because they are accustomed to their current setup, even if it's less safe.

Explanation: People naturally gravitate towards routines and familiar practices. Changes that disrupt these routines, even if they lead to improvements, can be met with resistance simply because they require effort to adapt.

Example: Employees might prefer sticking to their old, unsafe habits because they find it easier than learning and adjusting to new procedures.

10. Inadequate Resources

Illustration: Workers at a construction site might resist new safety gear requirements if the company does not provide sufficient or appropriate equipment.

Explanation: Employees are more likely to resist changes if they feel they do not have the necessary resources or support to comply. This includes adequate training, equipment, and time to adapt to new procedures.

Example: Employees might resist using new safety equipment if it is uncomfortable or not readily available.

11. Perceived Irrelevance

Illustration: Staff in a corporate office might resist fire drill protocols if they believe the risk of a fire is negligible.

Explanation: If employees perceive the new safety measures as irrelevant or unnecessary for their specific context, they are likely to resist them. Ensuring that the rationale for changes is clearly communicated and directly related to their work environment can help mitigate this resistance.

Example: Office workers might resist participating in regular emergency evacuation drills because they believe it's a waste of time given their low-risk environment.

To address these various forms of resistance, organizations should:

Build Trust: Foster open communication and transparency to build trust between leadership and employees.

Leverage Past Learnings: Acknowledge past failures and demonstrate how new changes address previous shortcomings.

Provide Clear Information: Ensure comprehensive, accessible information is provided to all employees.

Reassure Job Security: Clearly communicate that safety changes are not linked to job cuts but to overall well-being.

Combat Peer Pressure: Create a culture that values safety and recognizes adherence to protocols.

Facilitate Adaptation: Support employees in adapting to new routines with adequate training and resources.

Ensure Relevance: Tailor safety measures to be directly applicable to specific roles and contexts.

Inability for Communicating Effectively may be a cause of unsafe conditions.: Provide communication strategies for addressing resistance, including transparency, empathy, and active listening.

By understanding and addressing these diverse reasons for resistance, organizations can create a more supportive environment for implementing safety-related changes.

Important approaches:

Clear Communication:

Explanation: Clearly explain the reasons for the new safety measures, including the benefits and how they will protect employees and improve their work environment.

Action: Hold informational sessions and provide detailed documentation about the changes.

Involvement in the Change Process:

Explanation: Involve employees in the planning and implementation of safety changes to give them a sense of ownership and control.

Action: Create safety committees with employee representatives who can provide input and feedback.

Training and Education:

Explanation: Provide comprehensive training to ensure that employees feel competent and confident in the new procedures.

Action: Organize hands-on workshops and training sessions to familiarize employees with the new protocols.

Support Systems:

Explanation: Offer support to help employees transition to new safety measures, addressing their concerns and fears.

Action: Establish mentoring programs where experienced employees can help their peers adapt to changes.

Highlighting Benefits:

Explanation: Emphasize the long-term benefits of the new safety measures, such as reduced injury rates and a safer work environment.

Action: Share success stories and data from other organizations that have successfully implemented similar changes.

Addressing Practical Concerns:

Explanation: Address any practical concerns or inconveniences associated with the new safety measures by seeking input and making adjustments as necessary.

Action: Pilot the new procedures in small groups and refine them based on feedback before a full-scale rollout.

By understanding and addressing the specific reasons for resistance to safety-related changes, organizations can more effectively implement new safety protocols and create a safer, more cooperative work environment.

3.1.2 Communicating Effectively: Provide communication strategies for addressing resistance, including transparency, empathy, and active listening.

Effective communication is essential for overcoming resistance to safety-related changes. Below are key strategies that can help address resistance by fostering understanding, trust, and collaboration:

1. Transparency

Explanation: Transparency involves openly sharing information about the reasons behind safety changes, the expected benefits, and the processes involved. This helps to build trust and reduce uncertainty.

Strategies:

Detailed Briefings: Conduct regular meetings or briefings to explain the need for new safety protocols and how they will be implemented.

Open Forums: Create opportunities for employees to ask questions and receive honest answers. This can be done through town hall meetings, Q&A sessions, or online forums.

Regular Updates: Keep employees informed about the progress of the safety initiatives, any changes to the plan, and the results of implemented measures.

Example: A company implementing a new chemical handling procedure might hold a series of informational meetings explaining the dangers of improper handling, how the new procedures mitigate these dangers, and what steps are being taken to ensure everyone's safety.

2. Empathy

Explanation: Empathy involves understanding and acknowledging employees' feelings and concerns about safety changes. By showing empathy, leaders can build a stronger connection with their teams and address their worries more effectively.

Strategies:

One-on-One Conversations: Engage in personal conversations with employees to understand their specific concerns and fears about the new safety measures. Acknowledging Concerns: Validate employees' feelings by acknowledging that their concerns are legitimate and important. Providing Support: Offer resources such as counseling, peer support groups, or additional training to help employees cope with changes.

Example: If employees express fear about using new machinery, leaders could organize small group meetings where workers can voice their concerns and receive assurances about the extensive training and support that will be provided.

3. Active Listening

Explanation: Active listening is the process of fully concentrating, understanding, responding, and remembering what employees are saying. This approach helps to ensure that their concerns are heard and addressed appropriately.

Strategies:

Reflective Listening: Repeat or paraphrase what the employee has said to show that you have heard and understood their concerns.

Non-Verbal Cues: Use positive body language, such as nodding and maintaining eye contact, to show that you are engaged in the conversation.

Follow-Up: After initial conversations, follow up with employees to demonstrate that their feedback has been taken seriously and to provide updates on any actions taken in response.

Example: During a discussion about a new safety protocol, a supervisor might say, "I hear that you're worried about how this will impact your daily tasks. Can you tell me more about specific aspects that concern you?"

Implementing the Strategies

Create a Communication Plan: Develop a comprehensive plan that outlines how and when information will be communicated, who will deliver it, and what channels will be used (e.g., email, meetings, newsletters). Training for Leaders: Provide training for supervisors and managers on effective communication techniques, including how to demonstrate transparency, empathy, and active listening.

Feedback Mechanisms: Establish feedback mechanisms such as suggestion boxes, surveys, or digital platforms where employees can voice their concerns and suggestions anonymously if they prefer.

Visual Aids: Use visual aids such as posters, infographics, and videos to reinforce key messages and make information more accessible.

Celebrate Milestones: Recognize and celebrate milestones in the implementation of safety measures to maintain momentum and show appreciation for employees' cooperation and contributions.

By integrating these communication strategies, organizations can effectively address resistance to safety-related changes, fostering a safer and more cooperative work environment.

3.1.3 Engaging Stakeholders: Discuss the importance of involving employees in the change process and soliciting their input to mitigate resistance and increase buy-in.

Engaging Employees as Important Stakeholders

Involving employees as key stakeholders in the change process is crucial for mitigating resistance and increasing buy-in. When employees feel valued and included in decision-making, they are more likely to support and actively participate in safety initiatives. Here are key reasons and strategies for engaging employees effectively:

Importance of Employee Involvement

Ownership and Accountability: When employees are involved in the change process, they are more likely to take ownership and hold themselves accountable for the success of safety initiatives.

Diverse Perspectives: Employees bring a variety of perspectives and insights that can identify potential challenges and innovative solutions that management might overlook.

Enhanced Trust and Morale: Involving employees in the decision-making process fosters trust and improves morale, as they feel their opinions and contributions are valued.

Reduced Resistance: When employees understand the reasons behind changes and have a say in how they are implemented, resistance decreases as they feel part of the solution rather than the target of changes.

Strategies for Engaging Employees

Inclusive Decision-Making

Explanation: Involve employees at all levels in discussions about safety changes. This can be done through committees, focus groups, or cross-functional teams.

Example: Form a safety committee with representatives from different departments to gather input on new safety protocols and to discuss potential improvements.

Soliciting Feedback

Explanation: Regularly ask for employees' feedback on proposed safety measures and current practices. Use surveys, suggestion boxes, or digital platforms to collect input.

Example: Conduct an anonymous survey to gather opinions on new safety equipment or procedures before implementation, ensuring all voices are heard.

Regular Communication

Explanation: Keep employees informed about the progress and impact of safety initiatives. Use multiple communication channels such as newsletters, emails, meetings, and digital platforms.

Example: Hold monthly safety meetings where updates are provided, feedback is reviewed, and employees can ask questions or raise concerns.

Training and Education

Explanation: Provide training sessions that not only educate employees on new safety procedures but also solicit their input on how these procedures can be improved or better implemented.

Example: During a training session on new machinery, ask employees for their suggestions on additional safety measures or tips on using the equipment effectively.

Empowerment and Recognition

Explanation: Empower employees to take initiative in identifying and solving safety issues. Recognize and reward those who contribute positively to safety initiatives.

Example: Implement a "Safety Champion" program where employees who identify potential hazards or contribute to improving safety measures are publicly recognized and rewarded.

Collaborative Problem-Solving

Explanation: Encourage collaborative problem-solving sessions where employees work together to identify safety risks and develop solutions.

Example: Organize workshops where employees can brainstorm ideas for improving workplace safety and then collaborate to develop action plans.

Feedback Loops

Explanation: Establish feedback loops to ensure that employees know their input has been heard and acted upon. This can involve regular updates on the status of suggestions or changes based on their feedback.

Example: After receiving feedback through a survey, provide a detailed response outlining which suggestions will be implemented, the timeline for changes, and any additional steps being taken.

Implementing the Strategies

Establish a Structured Process: Develop a structured process for involving employees in safety initiatives, including regular meetings, surveys, and feedback sessions.

Leadership Commitment: Ensure that organizational leaders are committed to involving employees and are visibly supportive of employee input and participation.

Communication Plan: Create a comprehensive communication plan that outlines how employee involvement will be communicated and how feedback will be addressed.

Recognition Programs: Develop recognition programs that reward employees for their contributions to safety improvements and encourage ongoing participation.

Continuous Improvement: Foster a culture of continuous improvement where employee feedback is regularly solicited, and changes are made based on this input to enhance safety.

By engaging employees as important stakeholders, organizations can build a collaborative and inclusive culture that supports safety initiatives and reduces resistance to change. This approach not only enhances safety outcomes but also strengthens overall employee engagement and satisfaction.

Similarly other stakeholders need to be engaged in the right spirit to minimize occurrences of unusual incidents which can largely enhance productivity.

3.2 CHANGING NEGATIVE ATTITUDES

Overcoming Attitude Barriers: Changing Negative Attitudes

Changing negative attitudes towards safety is essential for creating a culture of safety within any organization. Negative attitudes can undermine safety initiatives, increase the risk of accidents, and reduce overall morale. Addressing and transforming these attitudes requires a multifaceted approach that involves challenging assumptions, providing education, and offering robust support mechanisms.

Needs for Changing Negative Attitudes

Improving Safety Compliance: Negative attitudes can lead to non-compliance with safety protocols. Changing these attitudes encourages adherence to safety standards and reduces the likelihood of accidents and injuries.

Enhancing Workplace Morale: Negative attitudes often contribute to a toxic work environment. Transforming these attitudes can improve overall workplace morale, making the work environment more positive and productive.

Boosting Productivity: Positive attitudes towards safety can lead to more efficient and effective work practices, as employees are more likely to follow procedures and avoid disruptions caused by accidents.

Reducing Costs: Negative attitudes that lead to unsafe behaviors can result in significant costs due to accidents, injuries, and potential legal issues. Changing these attitudes can help reduce these costs.

Fostering a Safety Culture: A culture of safety requires collective positive attitudes towards safety. Changing negative attitudes is crucial for fostering a culture where safety is prioritized and valued by everyone.

Strategies for Changing Negative Attitudes

Challenging Assumptions

Explanation: Encourage individuals to question and reassess their negative beliefs and assumptions about safety. This can help them recognize the importance and benefits of positive safety attitudes.

Example: Conduct workshops that challenge common myths and misconceptions about safety, providing factual information and real-life examples to shift perspectives.

Providing Education and Awareness

Explanation: Offer educational programs and awareness campaigns that highlight the consequences of negative attitudes and the benefits of positive safety behaviors.

Example: Implement a safety awareness campaign that includes training sessions, posters, and informational materials showcasing the impact of positive safety attitudes on reducing workplace accidents.

Offering Support and Resources

Explanation: Provide support mechanisms such as counseling services, peer support groups, and employee assistance programs to help individuals overcome negative attitudes and develop more positive outlooks.

Example: Establish a peer mentoring program where employees with positive safety attitudes mentor those struggling with negative attitudes, offering guidance and support.

Encouraging Positive Reinforcement

Explanation: Use positive reinforcement to encourage and reward positive safety behaviors and attitudes. This can help shift negative attitudes by associating positive behaviors with tangible rewards.

Example: Create a recognition program that rewards employees who consistently demonstrate positive safety attitudes and behaviors with incentives such as bonuses, awards, or public recognition.

Facilitating Open Communication

Explanation: Foster an environment where open communication about safety concerns and attitudes is encouraged. This can help identify negative attitudes early and address them constructively.

Example: Hold regular safety meetings where employees can openly discuss their concerns, share their experiences, and suggest improvements without fear of retribution.

Role Modeling by Leadership

Explanation: Leaders should model positive safety attitudes and behaviors, setting an example for employees to follow. Seeing leaders prioritize safety can inspire employees to adopt similar attitudes.

Example: Ensure that leaders actively participate in safety initiatives, such as safety audits or training sessions, demonstrating their commitment to safety.

Creating a Supportive Environment

Explanation: Build a supportive workplace culture where employees feel comfortable seeking help and sharing their concerns. This can reduce negative attitudes by fostering a sense of community and mutual support.

Example: Develop a buddy system where new employees are paired with experienced colleagues who can offer support and guidance on safety practices and attitudes.

By addressing and changing negative attitudes towards safety, organizations can significantly enhance their safety culture, reduce accidents and injuries, and create a more positive and productive work environment. This requires a concerted effort involving education, support, communication, and leadership commitment to foster positive attitudes and behaviors.

3.2.1 Challenging Assumptions: Encourage individuals to challenge their own negative assumptions and beliefs about safety through self-reflection and open-mindedness.

Encouraging individuals to challenge their own negative assumptions and beliefs about safety is a critical step in fostering a culture of safety within any organization. This process involves promoting self-reflection and open-mindedness, encouraging individuals to question the validity of their beliefs and consider alternative perspectives. By challenging assumptions, individuals can gain a deeper understanding of the reasons behind their attitudes towards safety and identify opportunities for growth and change.

Self-reflection plays a key role in this process, as it allows individuals to examine their beliefs and behaviors in relation to safety. By taking the time to reflect on past experiences, personal values, and external influences, individuals can gain insight into the origins of their attitudes and identify any underlying biases or misconceptions. Open-mindedness is also essential, as it enables individuals to consider new information and perspectives that may challenge their existing beliefs. By remaining open to feedback and willing to reevaluate their assumptions, individuals can overcome resistance to change and adopt more positive attitudes towards safety. Through this process of self-reflection and open-mindedness, individuals can begin to challenge their negative assumptions and beliefs about safety, paving the way for a culture of safety built on trust, accountability, and continuous improvement.

Let us consider an example of an employee who has developed a negative attitude towards wearing personal protective equipment (PPE) on the job. This employee may believe that PPE is uncomfortable, inconvenient, and unnecessary for their specific tasks. As a result, they resist wearing PPE, putting themselves and others at risk of injury.

To address this resistance, the employee can engage in self-reflection by considering why they hold this belief and how it may impact their safety and the safety of those around them. They may reflect on past incidents or near misses where PPE could have prevented injury, as well as their personal values and responsibilities as a member of the team.

Additionally, the employee can remain open-minded to feedback from colleagues, supervisors, and safety professionals who emphasize the importance of wearing PPE for their own protection. By considering alternative perspectives and new information, the employee may begin to challenge their negative assumptions about PPE and recognize its role in ensuring their safety on the job.

Through this process of self-reflection and open-mindedness, the employee can gradually overcome their resistance to wearing PPE and develop a more positive attitude towards safety. They may come to appreciate the value of PPE in mitigating workplace hazards and actively choose to comply with safety protocols for the benefit of themselves and their colleagues. This example illustrates how challenging assumptions through self-reflection and open-mindedness can lead to positive changes in attitude and behavior towards safety.

3.2.2 Providing Education and Awareness: Offer educational resources and awareness campaigns to help individuals understand the consequences of negative attitudes and behaviors.

Providing education and awareness is essential for helping individuals understand the consequences of negative attitudes and behaviors towards safety. This involves offering various educational resources and organizing awareness campaigns tailored to address specific safety concerns and challenges within the workplace.

One way to provide education is through interactive training sessions, workshops, or seminars that cover topics related to safety attitudes and behaviors. These sessions can include discussions, case studies, and practical demonstrations to help individuals grasp the importance of adopting positive attitudes towards safety.

Additionally, educational materials such as brochures, posters, videos, and online modules can be distributed to employees to reinforce key safety messages and encourage reflection on their attitudes and behaviors. These materials should be informative, engaging, and accessible to all members of the workforce.

Awareness campaigns play a crucial role in promoting a culture of safety by raising awareness of potential hazards, reinforcing safety protocols, and highlighting the importance of positive attitudes. These campaigns can take various forms, such as safety awareness weeks, themed events, or safety challenges, designed to capture employees' attention and encourage active participation.

By providing education and awareness opportunities, organizations empower individuals to make informed decisions about their safety and develop a deeper understanding of the consequences of negative attitudes and behaviors. This proactive approach fosters a culture of safety where employees are motivated to prioritize safety in their daily activities and contribute to a safer work environment for everyone.

3.2.3 Offering Support and Resources: Provide support mechanisms such as counseling services, peer support groups, and employee assistance programs to help individuals overcome negative attitudes and develop more positive outlooks.

Offering support and resources is crucial for helping individuals overcome negative attitudes and develop more positive outlooks towards safety. This involves implementing various support mechanisms within the organization to address the root causes of negative attitudes and provide individuals with the assistance they need to make positive changes.

One important support mechanism is providing access to counseling services for employees who may be struggling with mental health issues or personal challenges that affect their attitude towards safety. Counseling sessions can provide individuals with a safe space to discuss their concerns, explore coping strategies, and receive guidance on how to manage stress and anxiety effectively.

Peer support groups are another valuable resource for individuals dealing with negative attitudes towards safety. These groups provide a platform for employees to connect with their peers who may have similar experiences and share advice, encouragement, and support. By fostering a sense of community and solidarity, peer support groups can help individuals feel less isolated and more motivated to make positive changes.

Employee assistance programs (EAPs) are comprehensive support programs that offer a wide range of services to help employees address personal and professional challenges that may impact their well-being and performance.

These programs often include counseling services, financial assistance, legal advice, and referrals to external resources, providing employees with holistic support to overcome negative attitudes and improve their overall quality of life.

By offering support and resources such as counseling services, peer support groups, and employee assistance programs, organizations demonstrate their commitment to the well-being of their employees and create a supportive environment where individuals feel valued, understood, and empowered to overcome negative attitudes towards safety.

This proactive approach not only benefits individual employees but also contributes to a positive safety culture and improved organizational performance.

3.3 CULTIVATING RESILIENCE

Cultivating resilience is essential for overcoming barriers to developing a positive attitude towards safety in the workplace.

Resilience refers to the ability to bounce back from challenges, setbacks, and adversity, and it plays a crucial role in helping individuals navigate obstacles and maintain a positive mindset despite difficulties.

One of the key reasons why cultivating resilience is important is that it enables individuals to cope more effectively with the various barriers they may encounter in their efforts to adopt a positive attitude towards safety. Whether facing resistance to change, negative attitudes from colleagues, or personal challenges, resilient individuals are better equipped to overcome these obstacles and stay focused on their goals.

Moreover, cultivating resilience helps individuals build psychological strength and emotional stability, which are essential for maintaining a positive attitude over the long term. By developing resilience, individuals can bounce back more quickly from setbacks, learn from their experiences, and adapt to new circumstances, all of which contribute to a more resilient and positive approach to safety.

Additionally, cultivating resilience fosters a sense of empowerment and self-efficacy, which are essential for driving positive change. When individuals believe in their ability to overcome challenges and make a difference, they are more likely to take proactive steps towards improving safety and influencing others to do the same.

Overall, cultivating resilience is crucial for overcoming barriers to developing a positive attitude towards safety because it equips individuals with the tools and mindset needed to navigate challenges, maintain a positive outlook, and drive meaningful change in the workplace.

3.3.1 Building Mental Toughness: Discuss strategies for building resilience and coping skills to help individuals navigate challenges and setbacks in the workplace.

Building mental toughness is essential for individuals to effectively navigate challenges and setbacks in the workplace, especially when it comes to maintaining a positive attitude towards safety. Mental toughness enables individuals to persevere in the face of adversity, stay focused on their goals, and bounce back from setbacks stronger than before.

Few strategies for building mental toughness:

Developing a Growth Mindset: Encourage individuals to adopt a growth mindset, which involves viewing challenges as opportunities for growth and learning rather than as threats. Emphasize the importance of embracing challenges, persisting in the face of setbacks, and learning from failures.

Setting Realistic Goals: Help individuals set realistic and achievable goals related to safety performance. Break down larger goals into smaller, manageable tasks, and encourage individuals to focus on making progress one step at a time. Celebrate small victories along the way to maintain motivation and momentum.

Practicing Positive Self-Talk: Teach individuals to recognize and challenge negative self-talk and replace it with positive affirmations and encouragement. Encourage them to cultivate a resilient mindset by reframing challenges as opportunities, focusing on their strengths, and maintaining confidence in their ability to overcome obstacles.

Building Emotional Intelligence: Foster the development of emotional intelligence skills, such as self-awareness, self-regulation, empathy, and social skills. Help individuals identify and manage their emotions effectively, communicate assertively and empathetically with others, and build strong relationships based on trust and mutual respect.

Coping Strategies: Provide individuals with a toolbox of coping strategies to help them manage stress and adversity effectively. Encourage the use of relaxation techniques, mindfulness meditation, deep breathing exercises, and physical activity to reduce stress and promote emotional well-being.

Seeking Support: Emphasize the importance of seeking support from colleagues, supervisors, and mental health professionals when needed. Encourage individuals to reach out for help, share their concerns openly, and seek guidance and advice from trusted sources.

Learning from Setbacks: Encourage individuals to view setbacks as opportunities for learning and growth. Help them identify lessons learned from past experiences, reflect on what went well and what could be improved, and apply these insights to future challenges.

Visualization and Mental Rehearsal: Encourage individuals to visualize themselves successfully overcoming challenges and achieving their safety goals. By mentally rehearsing positive outcomes and visualizing themselves performing well in challenging situations, individuals can build confidence and resilience.

Maintaining a Healthy Lifestyle: Emphasize the importance of maintaining a healthy lifestyle to support mental and emotional well-being. Encourage individuals to prioritize adequate sleep, nutrition, exercise, and relaxation to enhance their resilience and coping abilities.

Developing Problem-Solving Skills: Help individuals develop strong problem-solving skills to effectively address safety challenges and find solutions to complex problems. Teach them to break problems down into manageable steps, consider alternative approaches, and seek input from others when needed.

Cultivating Optimism: Foster optimism and a positive outlook by highlighting progress, successes, and opportunities for growth. Encourage individuals to focus on what they can control, maintain a sense of hope and possibility, and approach challenges with a solution-focused mindset.

Building Social Support Networks: Support the development of strong social support networks within the workplace and community. Encourage individuals to connect with colleagues, friends, and family members who can provide encouragement, advice, and emotional support during difficult times.

By incorporating these strategies into daily lives, individuals can strengthen their mental toughness and resilience, enabling them to thrive in the face of adversity and maintain a positive attitude towards safety.

US Marines are known for their ability to balance risk-taking with safety considerations effectively. Here are some key lessons that can be learned from their approach:

Training and Preparedness: Marines undergo extensive training to develop the skills and mindset necessary to assess risks accurately and make informed decisions in high-pressure situations. This training instills discipline, situational awareness, and a commitment to safety protocols, ensuring that Marines are well-prepared to handle risks effectively.

Mission Focus: Marines prioritize mission accomplishment while also recognizing the importance of ensuring the safety and well-being of their fellow Marines. This mission-focused mindset helps them make risk assessments based on the potential impact on the overall mission objectives, balancing the need to take calculated risks with the imperative to minimize unnecessary danger.

Leadership and Accountability: Marine leaders play a crucial role in promoting a culture of safety and risk management within their units. They lead by example, emphasizing the importance of adhering to safety procedures and taking calculated risks when necessary. Leaders hold themselves and their subordinates accountable for safety-related decisions and actions, fostering a sense of responsibility and ownership among all Marines.

Adaptability and Flexibility: Marines are trained to adapt to changing circumstances and adjust their plans and tactics accordingly. This adaptability enables them to respond effectively to unexpected risks and challenges while maintaining a focus on achieving their objectives safely.

Continuous Improvement: After-action reviews (AARs) and lessons learned processes are integral components of Marine training and operations. Marines regularly evaluate their performance, identify areas for improvement, and implement changes to enhance safety and effectiveness. This commitment to continuous learning and improvement helps Marines refine their risk management skills and mitigate future risks more effectively.

Overall, the US Marine Corps' approach to balancing risk-taking and safety emphasizes training, mission focus, leadership, adaptability, and continuous improvement. By incorporating these principles into their operations, organizations in various sectors can enhance their risk management practices and achieve their objectives safely and effectively.

3.3.2 Promoting Work-Life Balance: Emphasize the importance of work-life balance in reducing stress and enhancing resilience and provide tips for managing workload and prioritizing self-care.

Promoting work-life balance is essential for reducing stress, enhancing resilience, and fostering overall well-being. Here are some tips for managing workload and prioritizing self-care to achieve a healthy balance:

Set Boundaries: Establish clear boundaries between work and personal life to prevent work from encroaching on your personal time. Define specific hours for work and stick to them as much as possible. Avoid checking work emails or taking work-related calls outside of these hours.

Prioritize Tasks: Identify the most important tasks and deadlines at work and prioritize them accordingly. Focus on completing high-priority tasks first, and delegate or defer less critical tasks when necessary. This helps prevent feeling overwhelmed and allows you to manage your workload more effectively.

Manage Time Wisely: Use time management techniques such as setting deadlines, breaking tasks into smaller, manageable chunks, and using tools like calendars and to-do lists to stay organized. Schedule regular breaks throughout the day to rest and recharge, helping to maintain productivity and reduce stress.

Practice Self-Care: Make self-care a priority by allocating time for activities that promote physical and mental well-being, such as exercise, meditation, hobbies, and spending time with loved ones. Engaging in activities you enjoy helps reduce stress, boost mood, and increase resilience in the face of challenges.

Communicate with Your Employer: If you're feeling overwhelmed with your workload or struggling to maintain work-life balance, don't hesitate to communicate with your employer or supervisor. Discuss any concerns or challenges you're facing and explore potential solutions together, such as adjusting deadlines, redistributing tasks, or implementing flexible work arrangements.

Set Realistic Expectations: Be realistic about what you can accomplish within a given timeframe and avoid overcommitting yourself. Learn to say no to additional responsibilities or projects when your plate is already full, and don't hesitate to ask for help or support when needed.

Unplug and Recharge: Take regular breaks from work, including evenings, weekends, and vacation time, to disconnect from work-related activities and focus on relaxation and rejuvenation. Engage in activities that help you recharge and unwind, whether it's spending time outdoors, reading a book, or pursuing a hobby.

Establish Rituals: Create rituals or routines that help you transition between work and personal life. This could include a morning routine to prepare for the workday and an evening routine to wind down and relax. Rituals can help signal to your brain that it's time to shift focus and can contribute to a sense of balance and stability.

Practice Mindfulness: Incorporate mindfulness practices into your daily routine to cultivate awareness and presence in the moment. Mindfulness techniques such as deep breathing exercises, meditation, or simply taking a few minutes to pause and observe your surroundings can help reduce stress, increase focus, and promote overall well-being.

Set Aside Time for Yourself: Carve out dedicated time for activities that nourish your soul and bring you joy. Whether it's pursuing a hobby, spending time with loved ones, or indulging in self-care activities like a relaxing bath or a leisurely walk in nature, prioritizing personal time is essential for maintaining balance and preventing burnout.

Delegate and Outsource: Don't hesitate to delegate tasks or responsibilities at work and at home when you're feeling overwhelmed. Identify tasks that can be outsourced or delegated to others, whether it's hiring a virtual assistant to handle administrative tasks or assigning household chores to family members. Delegating allows you to focus on high-priority activities and frees up time for activities that matter most to you.

Practice Gratitude: Cultivate a mindset of gratitude by reflecting on the things you're thankful for in both your professional and personal life. Keeping a gratitude journal or simply taking a few moments each day to acknowledge the positive aspects of your life can help shift your perspective, reduce stress, and foster a greater sense of balance and well-being.

Set Clear Work-Life Boundaries: Clearly define boundaries between work and personal life and communicate them to your colleagues, clients, and family members. Set expectations around when you're available for work-related matters and when you're off the clock. Respect your boundaries and encourage others to do the same, which helps prevent burnout and promotes a healthier work-life balance.

By incorporating these tips into daily routine, one can effectively manage workload, prioritize self-care, and achieve a healthier work-life balance, leading to reduced stress, increased resilience, and overall well-being.

3.3.3 Creating a Supportive Environment: Foster a supportive workplace culture where individuals feel comfortable seeking help, sharing concerns, and receiving encouragement from colleagues and leaders.

Creating a supportive environment in the workplace is essential for fostering employee well-being, collaboration, and overall success. Here's how organizations can cultivate a supportive culture:

Encourage Open Communication: Foster an environment where open communication is valued and encouraged. Encourage employees to share their ideas, concerns, and feedback without fear of judgment or reprisal. Leaders should lead by example by actively listening to employee input, addressing concerns promptly, and being transparent about organizational decisions and changes.

Provide Opportunities for Growth and Development: Support employee growth and development by providing opportunities for learning, training, and career advancement. Offer mentorship programs, professional development workshops, and access to resources that enable employees to enhance their skills and progress in their careers. Investing in employee development demonstrates a commitment to their success and well-being.

Promote Work-Life Balance: Recognize the importance of work-life balance and take steps to support employees in achieving it. Offer flexible work arrangements, such as remote work options or flexible scheduling, which accommodate employees' personal needs and obligations. Encourage employees to take breaks, use their vacation time, and prioritize self-care to prevent burnout and maintain overall well-being.

Foster a Sense of Belonging: Create a sense of belonging and inclusivity by celebrating diversity and fostering a culture of respect and acceptance. Encourage team building activities, social events, and initiatives that bring employees together and strengthen relationships. Promote a zero-tolerance policy for discrimination, harassment, and bullying, and take swift action to address any instances of misconduct.

Provide Supportive Leadership: Cultivate leadership styles that prioritize empathy, compassion, and support. Train managers and leaders to effectively support their teams, provide constructive feedback, and recognize employees' contributions. Encourage leaders to check in regularly with their team members, offer guidance and mentorship, and create opportunities for professional growth and advancement.

By creating a supportive environment where employees feel valued, respected, and empowered, organizations can foster a culture of collaboration, innovation, and success. This not only enhances employee satisfaction and retention but also contributes to overall organizational effectiveness and performance.

This chapter "Overcoming Attitude Barriers" explores the challenges individuals and organizations face when attempting to instigate change and foster positive safety attitudes. It begins by addressing Resistance to Change, exploring common reasons for resistance such as fear of the unknown, loss of control, and perceived inconvenience. Strategies for overcoming this resistance include effective communication techniques like transparency, empathy, and active listening, as well as engaging stakeholders to increase buy-in and mitigate resistance.

Moving on to Changing Negative Attitudes, the chapter emphasizes the importance of challenging assumptions and beliefs through self-reflection and open-mindedness. Providing Education and Awareness plays a pivotal role in this process, offering resources and campaigns to enlighten individuals about the consequences of negative attitudes and behaviors. Additionally, Offering Support and Resources, such as counseling services and peer support groups, aids in helping individuals overcome negativity and develop a more positive outlook towards safety.

Finally, Cultivating Resilience is explored as a means to navigate challenges and setbacks in the workplace. Building

Mental Toughness is discussed, outlining strategies for developing resilience and coping skills. Promoting Work-Life Balance is emphasized to reduce stress and enhance resilience, with tips provided for managing workload and prioritizing self-care. Creating a Supportive Environment is also highlighted as crucial, fostering a workplace culture where individuals feel supported, heard, and encouraged by their colleagues and leaders. Through these strategies, organizations can effectively overcome attitude barriers and cultivate a culture of safety and resilience.

A strong positive attitude will create more miracles than any wonder drug - Tony Robbins

As we conclude our exploration of overcoming attitude barriers, we transition seamlessly into Chapter 4, where the focus shifts towards integrating attitude-based safety into daily practices. Having addressed the various challenges and obstacles that hinder positive safety attitudes, Chapter 4 seeks to delve deeper into embedding safety within the organizational culture. By setting the tone at the top, establishing clear expectations, and creating mechanisms for accountability, organizations can foster an environment where safety becomes an inherent part of everyday operations.

Chapter 4 also emphasizes the importance of encouraging proactive safety behaviors among employees. Empowering individuals to take ownership of safety, promoting observation and reporting of hazards, and rewarding proactive actions are key strategies outlined in this section. By instilling a sense of responsibility and vigilance, organizations can create a culture where safety is everyone's priority. Finally, the chapter emphasizes the significance of fostering continuous improvement in safety practices. Learning from incidents, soliciting feedback from employees, and implementing iterative changes ensure that safety remains a dynamic and evolving aspect of organizational operations, driving towards ever-improving safety performance.

Chapter 4: Integrating Attitude-Based Safety into Daily Practices

Excellence is not an act, but a habit.

- Aristotle

4.1 EMBEDDING SAFETY IN ORGANIZATIONAL CULTURE

Embedding safety in organizational culture is about creating an environment where safety is a fundamental value shared by everyone, from top executives to frontline employees. This involves integrating safety into every aspect of the organization, ensuring it becomes a natural part of daily operations and decision-making processes. Let's delve into various ways and means to achieve this:

1. Leadership Commitment and Role Modeling

Leadership Commitment: For safety to be truly embedded in the organizational culture, leaders must demonstrate a visible and genuine commitment to safety. This means not just talking about safety, but actively participating in safety initiatives and prioritizing safety in decision-making processes. Leaders should consistently allocate resources to safety programs and ensure that safety is a key agenda item in meetings and strategic planning.

Role Modeling: Leaders set the tone for the entire organization. When they consistently model safe behaviors and attitudes, it sends a powerful message to all employees. For example, if leaders always wear appropriate personal protective equipment (PPE) and strictly follow safety protocols, it encourages employees to do the same. Leaders should also be visible in their participation in safety activities, such as safety audits and training sessions.

2. Clear Communication and Education

Clear Communication: Effective communication is essential for embedding safety in organizational culture. Safety expectations, policies, and procedures should be clearly communicated through multiple channels, such as meetings, emails, newsletters, and posters. Regular safety briefings and updates help keep safety at the forefront of everyone's mind.

Safety Education and Training: Ongoing education and training are crucial. This includes comprehensive onboarding safety training for new employees, as well as regular refresher courses and updates on new safety protocols. Interactive training methods, such as simulations and hands-on practice, can enhance understanding and retention. Ensuring that employees understand the reasons behind safety procedures helps them appreciate the importance of adhering to them.

3. Establishing Safety Expectations and Accountability

Setting Clear Expectations: Clearly defined safety expectations help employees understand their roles and responsibilities in maintaining a safe work environment.

These expectations should be communicated during onboarding and reinforced regularly. Employees should know what constitutes safe behavior and the standards they are expected to meet.

Creating Accountability: Accountability is key to maintaining a safety culture. Implement systems to hold individuals accountable for their safety behaviors. This could involve regular safety audits, incorporating safety metrics into performance evaluations, and establishing consequences for non-compliance. Accountability ensures that safety is taken seriously at all levels of the organization.

4. Encouraging Employee Involvement

Empowering Employees: Empower employees to take an active role in safety. Encourage participation in safety committees, suggestion programs, and safety audits. When employees are involved in developing and implementing safety initiatives, they are more likely to take ownership of safety in their daily tasks.

Recognizing and Rewarding Safe Behavior: Recognition programs that reward safe behavior can motivate employees to adhere to safety standards. Consider implementing monthly safety awards, public acknowledgment of safety contributions, and incentives for teams that meet safety goals. Recognition reinforces the importance of safety and encourages ongoing commitment.

5. Building a Supportive Environment

Promoting a Positive Safety Culture: Foster an environment where safety concerns can be raised without fear of reprisal. Encourage open communication where employees feel comfortable reporting hazards or near misses. A positive safety culture is built on trust and mutual respect, where everyone feels responsible for each other's safety.

Providing Resources and Support: Ensure employees have the resources they need to work safely, including appropriate PPE, well-maintained equipment, and access to safety information. Additionally, provide support through initiatives such as employee assistance programs, which can help address personal issues that may impact safety.

6. Continuous Improvement and Feedback

Learning from Incidents: Treat every safety incident as a learning opportunity. Conduct thorough investigations to understand root causes and implement corrective actions. Share lessons learned with the entire organization to prevent future occurrences and demonstrate a commitment to continuous improvement.

Soliciting and Using Feedback: Regularly seek feedback from employees on safety practices and procedures. Use this feedback to identify areas for improvement and make necessary adjustments. A feedback loop ensures that safety practices evolve and improve over time.

7. Integrating Safety into Daily Operations

Safety in Daily Activities: Embed safety into every aspect of daily operations. This can include daily safety briefings, routine safety checks, and integrating safety discussions into regular team meetings. When safety is a part of everyday activities, it becomes second nature.

Visual Reminders: Use visual aids such as posters, signs, and digital displays to reinforce safety messages. Visual reminders keep safety top of mind and provide quick references for safe practices.

By incorporating these strategies, organizations can create a robust safety culture where safety is a shared responsibility and a core organizational value. This ongoing effort requires continuous dedication and engagement from everyone in the organization.

4.1.1 Setting the Tone: Discuss the role of leadership in setting the tone for safety culture and modeling positive safety attitudes and behaviors.

Embedding safety in organizational culture starts at the top. Leadership's commitment to safety is crucial in setting the tone for the entire organization. Leaders not only influence policies and procedures but also model the attitudes and behaviors that shape the organizational culture. Here's how leaders can effectively set the tone for a strong safety culture:

Demonstrating Commitment

Visible Engagement in Safety Initiatives: Leaders must be visibly involved in safety initiatives. This means participating in safety meetings, attending training sessions, and being present during safety audits and inspections. For example, a CEO who personally participates in safety training sends a powerful message about the importance of safety to the entire organization.

Allocating Resources: Leaders demonstrate their commitment by allocating sufficient resources to safety programs. This includes funding for safety training, equipment, and technology. By prioritizing budget allocations for safety, leaders show that safety is a non-negotiable priority.

Setting Clear Safety Goals: Establishing clear, measurable safety goals is essential. Leaders should set ambitious yet achievable targets for safety performance and communicate these goals throughout the organization. Regularly reviewing and discussing progress towards these goals keeps safety at the forefront of organizational priorities.

Modeling Positive Safety Attitudes and Behaviors

Leading by Example: Leaders must consistently model the safety behaviors they expect from their employees. For instance, if a safety protocol requires wearing personal protective equipment (PPE), leaders should be the first to comply. When employees see leaders following safety protocols diligently, they are more likely to do the same.

Promoting a Just Culture: A just culture is one where employees feel safe to report safety concerns and near misses without fear of punishment. Leaders play a crucial role in fostering this environment by responding to reports constructively and focusing on learning and improvement rather than blame.

Communicating the Importance of Safety: Regular and consistent communication about safety underscores its importance. Leaders should use every opportunity to talk about safety, whether in formal meetings, casual conversations, or written communications. Sharing personal stories or experiences related to safety can also make the message more relatable and impactful.

Engaging with Employees

Open Door Policy: Leaders should maintain an open-door policy for safety concerns. Encouraging employees to voice their safety concerns directly to leadership helps build trust and ensures that potential issues are addressed promptly.

Recognizing and Rewarding Safe Behavior: Recognition programs that highlight and reward safe behavior can motivate employees to prioritize safety. Leaders should publicly acknowledge individuals and teams who demonstrate exceptional commitment to safety, thereby reinforcing the desired behaviors.

Soliciting Feedback: Actively seeking feedback from employees about safety practices and procedures is vital.

Leaders should encourage employees to provide suggestions for safety improvements and act on this feedback to show that it is valued.

Creating a Safety-First Mindset

Embedding Safety in Strategic Planning: Safety should be a core component of the organization's strategic planning. This means considering the safety implications of new projects, processes, and policies from the outset. By integrating safety into strategic decisions, leaders ensure it remains a central organizational value.

Continuous Learning and Improvement: Leaders should foster a culture of continuous learning and improvement in safety. This involves staying updated on best practices, adopting new safety technologies, and continuously reviewing and improving safety protocols. Regularly celebrating milestones and improvements in safety performance keeps the momentum going.

Real-World Example

Consider a manufacturing company where the leadership team has made safety their top priority. The CEO conducts monthly walk-throughs of the production floor, engages in conversations with employees about safety concerns, and ensures that every meeting agenda includes a discussion on safety performance. Additionally, the company has implemented a robust safety training program, and employees are regularly recognized for their contributions to improving workplace safety. This visible commitment from leadership fosters a strong safety culture where every employee feels responsible for maintaining a safe work environment.

In conclusion, leaders set the tone for safety culture by demonstrating commitment, modeling positive behaviors, engaging with employees, and embedding safety into every aspect of the organization. When leaders prioritize safety, it creates a ripple effect that permeates the entire organization, fostering a culture where safety is ingrained in daily operations and valued by all.

4.1.2 Establishing Clear Expectations: Outline expectations for safety behaviors and attitudes and communicate them consistently throughout the organization.

Establishing clear expectations for safety behaviors and attitudes is crucial in fostering a culture of safety within any organization. Clear expectations provide a foundation for consistent and safe practices, ensuring that every member of the organization understands their role in maintaining a safe work environment. Here's how to outline and communicate these expectations effectively:

Outlining Safety Behaviors and Attitudes

1. Develop Comprehensive Safety Policies and Procedures:

- **Written Guidelines:** Create detailed written guidelines that outline the expected safety behaviors and attitudes. These should cover everything from the use of personal protective equipment (PPE) to reporting unsafe conditions and procedures for handling emergencies.

- **Accessible Documentation:** Ensure that these guidelines are easily accessible to all employees, whether through an internal website, employee handbook, or posted in common areas.

2. Define Specific Safety Roles & Responsibilities:

- **Role-Based Expectations:** Clearly define what is expected of each role within the organization concerning safety. For example, the responsibilities of a machine operator will differ from those of a supervisor or safety officer.

- **Accountability:** Assign accountability by specifying who is responsible for monitoring, enforcing, and adhering to safety protocols.

3. Establish Behavioral Standards:

- **Positive Attitudes:** Emphasize the importance of maintaining a positive attitude towards safety. This includes being proactive in identifying hazards, participating in safety training, and encouraging others to follow safety protocols.

- **Safe Practices:** Outline specific safe practices such as proper lifting techniques, adherence to lockout/tagout procedures, and the correct use of machinery and equipment.

4. Set Measurable Safety Goals:

- **Performance Metrics:** Establish clear, measurable safety goals such as reducing the number of incidents, increasing near-miss reporting, and improving compliance with safety training.

- **Continuous Improvement:** Encourage continuous improvement by regularly reviewing and updating safety goals based on performance metrics and feedback.

Communicating Safety Expectations

1. Consistent Messaging:

- **Regular Communication:** Use multiple communication channels to consistently reinforce safety expectations. This can include emails, newsletters, bulletin boards, and digital displays.

- **Leadership Involvement:** Ensure that leaders at all levels regularly communicate the importance of safety and model the expected behaviors.

2. Safety Training Programs:

- **Comprehensive Training:** Implement comprehensive safety training programs that cover all aspects of safety behavior and attitude. This training should be mandatory for all employees and tailored to specific roles.

- **Ongoing Education:** Offer refresher courses and ongoing education to keep safety practices and expectations fresh in employees' minds.

3. Visual Reminders:

- **Signage and Posters:** Use signage and posters strategically placed throughout the workplace to remind employees of key safety practices and attitudes.

- **Digital Reminders:** Utilize screens and digital boards to display safety messages, reminders, and updates.

4. Employee Involvement:

- **Feedback Mechanisms:** Create channels for employees to provide feedback on safety expectations and practices. This can include suggestion boxes, surveys, and regular safety meetings.

- **Inclusive Development:** Involve employees in the development and revision of safety policies and procedures to ensure they are practical and relevant.

5. Recognition and Reward Systems:

- **Acknowledge Compliance:** Regularly acknowledge and reward employees who consistently meet or exceed safety expectations. This can be through formal recognition programs, awards, or incentives.

- **Celebrate Success:** Celebrate milestones and achievements in safety performance to reinforce the importance of maintaining high safety standards.

6. Transparent Communication:

- **Open Dialogues:** Encourage open dialogue about safety issues and expectations. Hold regular meetings where employees can discuss safety concerns and suggest improvements.

- **Clear Consequences:** Communicate the consequences of not adhering to safety expectations clearly and fairly. Ensure that all employees understand the importance of compliance and the potential risks of non-compliance.

Example of Effective Communication:

At a large construction firm, the leadership team uses a multifaceted approach to communicate safety expectations. They have developed a comprehensive safety manual that is distributed to all employees. In addition, the company conducts monthly safety meetings where leaders discuss recent safety incidents, review procedures, and highlight employees who have demonstrated exemplary safety behaviors. Digital displays throughout the worksites provide constant reminders of key safety practices, and an open-door policy encourages employees to share their safety concerns and suggestions directly with management.

By establishing clear expectations and consistently communicating with them, organizations can create a unified approach to safety that empowers all employees to take responsibility for their own safety and the safety of their colleagues. This not only helps prevent accidents and injuries but also fosters a culture where safety is valued and prioritized every day.

4.1.3 Creating Accountability: Implement mechanisms for holding individuals accountable for their safety attitudes and behaviors, such as performance evaluations and recognition programs.

Creating accountability for safety attitudes and behaviors is essential to ensuring that all members of an organization take responsibility for maintaining a safe work environment.

By implementing robust mechanisms for accountability, organizations can reinforce the importance of safety, encourage compliance, and recognize positive contributions. Here's how to establish effective accountability systems:

Implementing Performance Evaluations

1. Integrate Safety into Performance Reviews:

- **Safety Metrics:** Incorporate safety metrics into regular performance evaluations. Assess employees on their adherence to safety protocols, participation in safety training, and proactive identification of hazards.

- **Behavioral Assessments:** Evaluate employees not just on safety compliance but also on their attitudes towards safety. This includes their willingness to follow procedures, report incidents, and encourage others to maintain safe practices.

2. Set Clear Safety Objectives:

- **Individual Goals:** Establish clear, measurable safety objectives for each employee based on their role. For example, a warehouse worker might have goals related to proper lifting techniques and reporting near-misses, while a manager might have objectives tied to conducting regular safety inspections and fostering a safety culture.

- **Regular Check-Ins:** Conduct regular check-ins to review progress towards these safety objectives. Provide constructive feedback and adjust goals as necessary to ensure continuous improvement.

3. Utilize 360-Degree Feedback:

- **Peer Reviews:** Implement 360-degree feedback systems where employees can provide input on their peers' safety attitudes and behaviors. This holistic approach can uncover areas for improvement and highlight positive contributions that might be overlooked by supervisors alone.

- **Self-Assessments:** Encourage employees to conduct self-assessments of their safety behaviors and attitudes. This reflective practice helps individuals recognize their strengths and areas for growth.

Recognition Programs

1. Formal Recognition Systems:

- **Safety Awards:** Develop formal recognition systems such as monthly or quarterly safety awards. Recognize individuals or teams who consistently demonstrate exemplary safety practices and attitudes.

- **Certificates and Plaques:** Provide tangible rewards like certificates, plaques, or trophies to acknowledge outstanding safety contributions. Display these awards in prominent areas to motivate others.

2. Incentive Programs:

- **Monetary Rewards:** Offer monetary incentives such as bonuses or gift cards for employees who meet or exceed safety expectations. These rewards can be tied to specific achievements like zero incidents for a quarter or exemplary safety leadership.

- **Non-Monetary Incentives:** Implement non-monetary incentives such as extra time off, preferred parking spots, or company merchandise. These rewards can also be effective in encouraging a positive safety culture.

3. Public Acknowledgment:

- **Company Newsletters:** Highlight safety achievements in company newsletters or internal communications. Share stories of employees who have gone above and beyond in promoting safety.

- **Meetings and Events:** Recognize safety champions during company meetings or events. Public acknowledgment reinforces the importance of safety and motivates others to follow suit.

Example of Accountability Mechanisms

In a manufacturing plant, the leadership team has implemented a comprehensive accountability system for safety. Employees undergo bi-annual performance reviews that include specific safety criteria, such as adherence to PPE usage and participation in safety drills. Additionally, the plant has a "Safety Star" program where employees can nominate their peers for monthly safety awards.

Winners receive a certificate, a gift card, and recognition during the monthly all-hands meeting. This combination of performance evaluations and recognition programs has significantly enhanced the plant's overall safety culture.

By establishing clear mechanisms for accountability, organizations can ensure that safety remains a top priority at all levels. These systems not only identify and address areas for improvement but also celebrate and reinforce positive safety behaviors and attitudes.

This balanced approach helps create a workplace where everyone feels responsible for and committed to maintaining a safe environment.

Encouraging Proactive Safety Behaviors: 10 Effective Strategies

1. Empowerment Through Education:

- **Comprehensive Training Programs:** Offer ongoing safety training that goes beyond basic compliance. Provide advanced courses on risk assessment, emergency response, and ergonomics to empower employees with in-depth knowledge.

- **Certifications and Workshops:** Encourage employees to obtain safety certifications and attend workshops. This not only enhances their skills but also fosters a culture of continuous learning and improvement.

2. Fostering Open Communication:

- **Safety Communication Channels:** Establish dedicated communication channels for safety-related discussions, such as a safety hotline or an online portal. Ensure these channels are accessible and promoted throughout the organization.

- **Regular Safety Meetings:** Hold regular safety meetings where employees can discuss concerns, share ideas, and suggest improvements. These meetings should be inclusive, allowing all voices to be heard.

3. Incentivizing Safety Participation:

- **Safety Incentive Programs:** Implement incentive programs that reward proactive safety behaviors. Offer bonuses, gift cards, or other rewards for reporting hazards, suggesting safety improvements, or demonstrating excellent safety practices.

- **Recognition and Awards:** Create recognition programs to celebrate safety champions. Monthly or quarterly awards can highlight employees who have gone above and beyond in promoting a safe work environment.

4. Engaging Safety Committees:

- **Employee-Led Safety Committees:** Form safety committees that include employees from various levels and departments. These committees can identify risks, develop solutions, and promote safety initiatives.

- **Committee Training:** Provide committee members with specialized training to enhance their ability to lead safety initiatives and influence their peers.

5. Promoting Observation and Reporting:

- **Near-Miss Reporting Systems:** Establish a robust system for reporting near-misses and potential hazards. Ensure that all reports are taken seriously and addressed promptly.

- **Safety Observation Programs:** Encourage employees to conduct safety observations and audits.

Train them to identify risks and provide constructive feedback to their colleagues.

6. Facilitating Employee Involvement:

- **Safety Suggestion Boxes:** Place suggestion boxes in common areas where employees can anonymously submit safety concerns or improvement ideas.

- **Engagement Surveys:** Conduct regular safety engagement surveys to gather employee feedback on safety practices and areas for improvement.

7. Leadership Support:

- **Visible Leadership Commitment:** Ensure that leaders visibly support and participate in safety initiatives. Their involvement sends a powerful message about the importance of safety.

- **Mentorship Programs:** Pair employees with safety mentors who can guide them in adopting and promoting safe behaviors.

8. Integrating Safety into Daily Operations:

- **Safety Moments:** Start meetings with a "safety moment" where a brief safety tip or incident review is discussed. This keeps safety at the forefront of daily operations.

- **Safety Checklists:** Use safety checklists for daily tasks to ensure that safety considerations are integrated into every aspect of work.

9. Leveraging Technology:

- **Safety Apps:** Utilize mobile apps that allow employees to report hazards, access safety information, and receive real-time updates.

- **Data Analytics:** Implement data analytics tools to monitor safety trends and identify areas for improvement. Use this data to inform proactive safety measures.

10. Creating a Safety-Focused Environment:

- **Safety Signage and Reminders:** Place safety signs, posters, and reminders throughout the workplace to reinforce safe practices and behaviors.

- **Workstation Ergonomics:** Ensure that workstations are ergonomically designed to minimize risk and promote safe work habits. Regularly review and adjust setups as needed.

By implementing these strategies, organizations can foster a proactive safety culture where employees feel empowered, engaged, and committed to maintaining a safe work environment.

4.2.1 Empowering Employees: Empower employees to take ownership of safety by providing training, resources, and opportunities for participation in safety initiatives.

Empowering Employees to Take Ownership of Safety

1. Comprehensive Training Programs:

- **Foundational Safety Training:** Start with a solid foundation. Provide new employees with thorough safety training during their onboarding process. This training should cover basic safety protocols, emergency procedures, and the organization's safety culture.

- **Advanced Training Opportunities:** Offer ongoing training opportunities to deepen employees' safety knowledge. This could include specialized courses in areas like hazardous materials handling, first aid, or fire safety. Advanced training helps employees feel more competent and confident in managing safety risks.

Example: A manufacturing company offers a series of training modules that employees can complete at their own pace. These modules cover everything from basic machine safety to advanced risk assessment techniques. Employees who complete all modules receive a certification and are recognized at company meetings.

2. Providing Resources:

- **Access to Safety Equipment:** Ensure that employees have easy access to the necessary safety equipment and personal protective equipment (PPE). Regularly inspect and maintain this equipment to guarantee its effectiveness.

- **Safety Literature and Manuals:** Distribute safety manuals and literature that employees can refer to when needed. This material should be clear, concise, and readily available in both digital and print formats.

Example: A construction firm provides all workers with a comprehensive safety handbook and ensures that all equipment is regularly inspected and maintained. They also have an online portal where employees can access safety resources, report issues, and find answers to common safety questions.

3. Opportunities for Participation:

- **Safety Committees:** Encourage employees to join safety committees. These committees can work on identifying potential hazards, suggesting improvements, and developing new safety initiatives. Committee members gain valuable experience and contribute directly to enhancing workplace safety.

- **Safety Champions Program:** Implement a Safety Champions program where employees volunteer or are nominated to act as safety advocates within their teams. These champions lead by example, promote safe practices, and serve as a point of contact for safety-related concerns.

Example: In a hospital setting, a Safety Champions program is established where nurses, doctors, and support staff can volunteer to lead safety initiatives. These champions conduct regular safety briefings, provide feedback on safety protocols, and ensure that their colleagues adhere to safety guidelines.

4. Encouraging Feedback and Involvement:

- **Suggestion Systems:** Set up a system for employees to submit safety suggestions and feedback. This can be an anonymous suggestion box or a digital platform. Act on this feedback to show employees that their input is valued and can lead to real change.

- **Regular Safety Meetings:** Hold regular safety meetings where employees can voice their concerns, share ideas, and discuss recent incidents or near-misses. These meetings should be inclusive, giving all employees a chance to participate.

Example: A retail company holds monthly safety meetings where employees can discuss recent safety incidents and near-misses. The company uses a digital suggestion box where employees can submit safety ideas anonymously. Each month, the best suggestions are implemented and recognized in the company newsletter.

5. Recognition and Rewards:

- **Incentive Programs:** Create incentive programs that reward employees for proactive safety behavior. This could include bonuses, gift cards, or other rewards for reporting hazards, participating in safety training, or demonstrating excellent safety practices.

- **Public Recognition:** Recognize employees who go above and beyond in promoting safety. This could be done through awards, certificates, or shout-outs during company meetings.

Example: An office environment introduces a "Safety Star" award, given monthly to an employee who has shown outstanding commitment to safety.

The award includes a certificate, a gift card, and a feature in the company newsletter.

By implementing these strategies, organizations can create an environment where employees feel empowered to take ownership of their safety.

This empowerment leads to a more engaged workforce, proactive safety behavior, and ultimately, a safer workplace.

4.2.2 Promoting Observation and Reporting: Encourage employees to actively observe their surroundings for safety hazards and to report near misses and safety concerns promptly.

Promoting Observation and Reporting in the Workplace

1. Creating a Culture of Vigilance:

- **Regular Safety Briefings:** Conduct regular safety briefings to remind employees of the importance of vigilance and staying alert to potential hazards. Use these briefings to highlight recent near misses and discuss how they were addressed.

- **Safety Awareness Campaigns:** Launch safety awareness campaigns that emphasize the importance of observation and reporting. Use posters, emails, and intranet updates to keep safety at the forefront of employees' minds.

Example: A manufacturing plant holds weekly safety briefings where supervisors discuss recent near misses and highlight the importance of reporting hazards. They also run a "See Something, Say Something" campaign with posters around the facility to encourage vigilance.

2. Training and Education:

- **Observation Skills Training:** Provide specific training on how to identify potential hazards in the workplace. Teach employees what to look for and how to assess different types of risks.

- **Reporting Procedures:** Ensure that all employees are familiar with the proper procedures for reporting hazards and near misses. This training should include how to use any reporting tools or forms the company uses.

Example: A construction company offers workshops on hazard identification where employees practice spotting potential risks on a mock construction site. They also provide clear instructions on how to report these hazards using a simple mobile app.

3. Simplifying the Reporting Process:

- **User-Friendly Reporting Tools:** Implement easy-to-use reporting tools, such as mobile apps or online forms, which allow employees to quickly and conveniently report hazards and near misses.

- **Anonymous Reporting Options:** Provide options for anonymous reporting to ensure that employees feel comfortable reporting issues without fear of retaliation.

Example: An office environment introduces a simple, user-friendly mobile app for reporting safety concerns and near misses. The app allows employees to submit reports anonymously if they choose.

4. Encouraging Immediate Action:

- **Quick Response Protocols:** Establish protocols for quickly addressing reported hazards. Ensure that reported issues are reviewed and acted upon promptly to demonstrate that employee concerns are taken seriously.

- **Feedback Loop:** Create a feedback loop where employees receive updates on the status of their reports and any actions taken. This transparency helps build trust and encourages continued reporting.

Example: In a healthcare facility, reported safety concerns are reviewed within 24 hours, and employees receive updates on the actions taken to address the issues. This quick response time shows employees that their reports lead to tangible improvements.

5. Recognition and Incentives:

- **Recognition Programs:** Recognize and reward employees who consistently observe and report safety hazards. This recognition can be in the form of certificates, public acknowledgments, or small rewards.

- **Incentive Programs:** Develop incentive programs that provide tangible rewards for proactive safety behaviors, such as gift cards, extra time off, or other perks.

Example: A logistics company runs a monthly "Safety Champion" program where employees who have reported hazards or near misses are recognized at company meetings and given a small gift card as a reward.

6. Promoting a No-Blame Culture:

- **Encouraging Reporting Without Fear:** Foster a culture where employees feel safe reporting hazards and near misses without fear of blame or punishment. Emphasize that the goal is to improve safety, not to assign blame.

- **Learning from Mistakes:** Use reported incidents as learning opportunities. Analyze near misses to identify root causes and implement preventative measures without focusing on individual fault.

Example: A chemical processing plant promotes a no-blame culture by using near-miss reports as case studies during safety meetings, focusing on what can be learned and how similar incidents can be prevented in the future.

7. Engaging Leadership:

- **Leadership Involvement:** Ensure that leaders at all levels are visibly involved in promoting safety observation and reporting. Leaders should model the desired behavior by actively participating in safety walks and reporting any hazards they observe.

- **Open Communication Channels:** Maintain open communication channels between employees and leadership, making it easy for employees to report concerns directly to their supervisors or safety managers.

Example: In a retail company, store managers regularly conduct safety walks with their teams, demonstrating the importance of vigilance. They also hold open office hours where employees can discuss safety concerns directly with them.

By implementing these strategies, organizations can create an environment where employees are proactive in observing and reporting safety hazards. This culture of vigilance and accountability leads to a safer workplace, as potential risks are identified and addressed before they result in accidents or injuries.

4.2.3 Rewarding Proactivity: Recognize and reward proactive safety behaviors through incentive programs, peer recognition, and public acknowledgment.

Rewarding Proactivity: Recognize and Reward Proactive Safety Behaviors

Recognizing and rewarding proactive safety behaviors is crucial to fostering a culture of safety in any organization. By acknowledging employees who actively contribute to a safer workplace, you not only motivate those individuals but also set a positive example for others to follow. Here are several strategies for effectively rewarding proactive safety behaviors:

1. Incentive Programs:

- **Safety Incentive Programs:** Implement structured safety incentive programs that reward employees for proactive safety behaviors. These programs can include points systems, where employees earn points for actions like reporting hazards or participating in safety drills, which can be redeemed for rewards.

- **Monetary Rewards:** Offer monetary rewards for employees who consistently demonstrate proactive safety behaviors. This could be in the form of bonuses, gift cards, or additional paid time off.

Example: A manufacturing company introduces a safety incentive program where employees earn points for reporting near misses, participating in safety training, and suggesting safety improvements. Points can be exchanged for gift cards or company merchandise.

2. Peer Recognition:

- **Safety Hero Awards:** Create a peer recognition program where employees can nominate their colleagues for "Safety Hero" awards. This encourages team members to recognize and appreciate each other's efforts in maintaining a safe workplace.

- **Peer-to-Peer Acknowledgment:** Encourage peer-to-peer acknowledgment through informal means, such as "safety shout-outs" during team meetings, where employees can publicly thank colleagues for their proactive safety actions.

Example: In a hospital, staff members can nominate their peers for a monthly "Safety Hero" award. Winners are featured in the hospital newsletter and receive a small token of appreciation, such as a certificate or a gift card.

3. Public Acknowledgment:

- **Safety Bulletin Boards:** Use safety bulletin boards in common areas to publicly acknowledge employees who have demonstrated proactive safety behaviors. Highlight their contributions and the positive impact they have had on workplace safety.

- **Company-Wide Announcements:** Recognize proactive safety behaviors through company-wide announcements, such as emails, newsletters, or intranet posts. Public acknowledgment reinforces the importance of safety and celebrates those who contribute to it.

Example: A construction company has a "Safety Star" board in the break room, where photos and descriptions of employees' proactive safety actions are posted. Additionally, these employees are highlighted in the company's monthly newsletter.

4. Recognition Ceremonies:

- **Annual Safety Awards:** Host an annual safety awards ceremony where employees are recognized for their contributions to workplace safety. Categories can include "Most Reports of Near Misses," "Best Safety Improvement Suggestion," and "Safety Role Model."

- **Quarterly Celebrations:** Hold quarterly safety celebrations where employees are acknowledged for their ongoing commitment to safety. These events can include presentations of awards, sharing success stories, and social activities.

Example: An energy company hosts an annual safety awards gala where employees are honored for their exceptional safety contributions. Awards include trophies, certificates, and special commendations from senior management.

5. Personalized Recognition:

- **Customized Rewards:** Tailor rewards the preferences of individual employees. Some may prefer public recognition, while others might appreciate private acknowledgment or personalized thank-you notes from leadership.

- **One-on-One Meetings:** Leaders can hold one-on-one meetings with employees to personally thank them for their proactive safety efforts and discuss the positive impact of their actions on the organization.

Example: A logistics company's safety manager sends personalized thank-you notes to employees who have gone above and beyond in their safety duties, highlighting specific actions and their outcomes.

By implementing these strategies, organizations can effectively recognize and reward proactive safety behaviors, fostering a culture where safety is prioritized and valued by all employees. This not only enhances overall safety but also promotes a sense of pride and responsibility among the workforces.

In addition to the strategies mentioned earlier, here are some more ways to create a proactive safety attitude in the workplace:

1. **Training and Education:** Provide comprehensive safety training programs that not only cover basic safety protocols but also emphasize the importance of proactive safety behaviors. Ensure that all employees understand potential hazards and know how to identify and address them proactively.

2. **Open Communication Channels:** Foster an environment where employees feel comfortable expressing safety concerns, sharing ideas for improvement, and reporting near misses without fear of reprisal. Encourage two-way communication between management and employees to ensure that safety issues are addressed promptly.

3. **Leadership Involvement:** Demonstrate visible support for safety initiatives from top leadership. When employees see that leaders prioritize safety and actively participate in safety-related activities, they are more likely to follow suit. Leaders should lead by example and consistently promote proactive safety behaviors.

4. **Continuous Improvement:** Encourage a culture of continuous improvement by regularly reviewing safety

processes, procedures, and protocols. Solicit feedback from employees on ways to enhance safety practices and implement necessary changes to address identified gaps or risks.

5. **Empowerment and Ownership:** Empower employees to take ownership of safety in their own work areas. Provide them with the authority and resources to address safety concerns proactively, whether it involves implementing safety improvements, conducting safety inspections, or leading safety training sessions for their peers.

6. **Safety Committees and Teams:** Establish safety committees or teams composed of representatives from different departments or work areas. These teams can collaborate on identifying safety hazards, developing solutions, and implementing proactive safety measures tailored to specific job tasks or work environments.

7. **Regular Safety Audits and Inspections:** Conduct regular safety audits and inspections to identify potential hazards and assess the effectiveness of existing safety controls. Encourage employees to actively participate in these audits and provide input on safety improvements.

8. **Recognition and Rewards:** Implement a formal system for recognizing and rewarding proactive safety behaviors. This can include incentives for reporting near misses, safety suggestion programs, or rewards for departments with exemplary safety records.

Recognizing and rewarding proactive safety efforts reinforces desired behaviors and motivates employees to remain vigilant about safety.

9. **Safety Culture Surveys:** Periodically conduct surveys or assessments to gauge the organization's safety culture and identify areas for improvement. Use the feedback obtained from these surveys to refine safety initiatives and tailor interventions to address specific challenges or concerns raised by employees.

10. **Leading Indicators:** Shift the focus from lagging indicators (e.g., injury rates) to leading indicators that measure proactive safety behaviors and safety performance. Monitor leading indicators such as near miss reporting rates, safety training participation, and safety observation data to track progress and identify areas for improvement in real-time.

By incorporating these additional elements into proactive safety initiatives, employers can further enhance safety awareness, engagement, and ownership throughout the organization, ultimately leading to a safer and healthier work environment for all employees.

4.3 Fostering Continuous Improvement

Fostering continuous improvement in safety practices and attitudes is crucial for maintaining a safe work environment. Here are 10 strategies to achieve this:

1. **Regular Safety Reviews:** Conduct regular reviews of safety policies, procedures, and practices to identify areas for improvement. Solicit feedback from employees, safety committees, and external safety experts to ensure that safety measures are effective and up to date.

2. **Incident Analysis:** Thoroughly investigate all safety incidents, including near misses, accidents, and injuries, to identify root causes and implement corrective actions. Use incident analysis as a learning opportunity to prevent similar incidents from occurring in the future.

3. **Training and Education:** Provide ongoing safety training and education for employees at all levels of the organization. Offer specialized training on topics such as hazard recognition, emergency response procedures, and safety best practices to ensure that employees have the knowledge and skills to work safely.

4. **Safety Culture Assessments:** Conduct regular assessments of the organization's safety culture to gauge employee attitudes, perceptions, and behaviors related to safety. Use the results of these assessments to identify strengths and weaknesses in the safety culture and develop targeted interventions to promote continuous improvement.

5. **Benchmarking and Best Practices:** Benchmark safety performance against industry standards and best practices to identify opportunities for improvement.

Learn from other organizations with strong safety records and adopt their successful strategies and initiatives.

6. **Employee Involvement:** Encourage active participation and involvement from employees in safety improvement initiatives. Empower employees to identify safety hazards, suggest improvements, and participate in decision-making processes related to safety.

7. **Safety Committees:** Establish safety committees or teams composed of representatives from different departments or work areas to oversee safety initiatives and drive continuous improvement efforts. Provide these committees with the authority and resources needed to implement safety improvements and monitor progress.

8. **Safety Performance Metrics:** Develop and track key safety performance metrics to measure progress and identify areas for improvement. Monitor leading indicators such as near misses, safety observations, and safety training completion rates to proactively identify potential safety risks and address them before they escalate.

9. **Continuous Communication:** Foster open and transparent communication channels related to safety throughout the organization. Encourage employees to report safety concerns, near misses, and hazards

promptly, and ensure that these reports are addressed in a timely manner.

10. **Management Commitment:** Demonstrate visible leadership commitment to safety by prioritizing safety initiatives, allocating resources for safety improvements, and actively participating in safety-related activities. Engage with employees at all levels of the organization to reinforce the importance of safety and promote a culture of continuous improvement.

By implementing these strategies, organizations can foster a culture of continuous improvement in safety practices and attitudes, ultimately leading to a safer and healthier work environment for all employees.

4.3.1 Learning from Incidents: Encourage a culture of learning from safety incidents and near misses by conducting thorough investigations and implementing corrective actions.

Learning from incidents and near misses is essential for improving safety practices and preventing future accidents. Here's how organizations can encourage a culture of learning from incidents:

1. **Thorough Investigations:** Conduct thorough investigations into safety incidents and near misses to understand the root causes and contributing factors. Involve all relevant stakeholders, including frontline workers, supervisors, and safety professionals, in the

investigation process to gather diverse perspectives and insights.

2. **Root Cause Analysis:** Use established root cause analysis techniques, such as the Five Whys or Fishbone Diagram, to systematically identify the underlying causes of safety incidents. Look beyond the immediate causes to uncover deeper organizational, procedural, or systemic issues that may have contributed to the incident.

3. **Documentation and Reporting:** Establish clear procedures for documenting and reporting safety incidents and near misses. Encourage employees to report incidents promptly and without fear of reprisal, emphasizing the importance of learning from mistakes to prevent future accidents.

4. **Sharing Lessons Learned:** Share the findings of incident investigations transparently with all employees, highlighting key lessons learned and recommendations for preventing similar incidents in the future. Use various communication channels, such as safety meetings, newsletters, or intranet platforms, to disseminate this information widely.

5. **Implementing Corrective Actions:** Develop and implement corrective actions based on the findings of incident investigations. Prioritize actions that address the root causes of incidents and focus on preventing recurrence. Assign responsibility for implementing and

monitoring corrective actions to specific individuals or teams to ensure accountability.

6. **Training and Awareness:** Provide training and awareness programs to educate employees about the lessons learned from incidents and near misses. Use real-life case studies and examples to illustrate the importance of identifying and mitigating safety hazards proactively.

7. **Continuous Improvement:** Use the insights gained from incident investigations to drive continuous improvement in safety practices and procedures. Regularly review and update safety policies, procedures, and training programs based on lessons learned from past incidents.

8. **Feedback Mechanisms:** Establish feedback mechanisms to gather input from employees on the effectiveness of corrective actions and the overall safety improvement process. Encourage employees to provide suggestions for further improvements and actively involve them in shaping the safety culture of the organization.

9. **Recognition and Reinforcement:** Recognize and reward individuals and teams that contribute to improving safety through their proactive efforts in incident investigation, corrective action implementation, and safety advocacy. Celebrate successes and milestones in the organization's journey towards a safer work environment.

10. **Leadership Commitment:** Demonstrate visible leadership commitment to learning from incidents and near misses by actively participating in incident investigations, supporting corrective action implementation, and reinforcing a culture of continuous improvement in safety. Leaders should lead by example and prioritize safety as a core value of the organization.

By promoting a culture of learning from incidents and near misses, organizations can proactively identify and address safety hazards, prevent accidents, and continuously improve their safety performance.

4.3.2 Soliciting Feedback: Seek feedback from employees on safety practices, procedures, and attitudes, and use this input to identify areas for improvement.

Soliciting feedback from employees is a crucial aspect of fostering a culture of safety and continuous improvement within an organization. Here's how organizations can effectively solicit feedback from their employees on safety practices, procedures, and attitudes:

1. **Anonymous Surveys:** Conduct regular anonymous surveys to gather feedback from employees on various aspects of safety within the organization. Use targeted questions to assess perceptions of safety culture, the effectiveness of safety training programs, and suggestions for improvement.

2. **Focus Groups:** Organize focus group discussions with representatives from different departments or job roles to delve deeper into specific safety issues or concerns. Encourage open and honest dialogue, allowing employees to share their perspectives and experiences freely.

3. **Safety Committees:** Establish safety committees comprised of representatives from management and frontline workers to serve as a forum for discussing safety-related matters and soliciting feedback. Empower these committees to review safety policies, procedures, and incident reports, and make recommendations for improvement.

4. **One-on-One Meetings:** Schedule regular one-on-one meetings between supervisors and their direct reports to discuss safety concerns, feedback, and suggestions for improvement. Create a supportive environment where employees feel comfortable raising safety-related issues without fear of reprisal.

5. **Anonymous Reporting Systems:** Implement anonymous reporting systems, such as suggestion boxes or online platforms, where employees can submit safety-related feedback or concerns confidentially. Ensure that these systems are easily accessible and user-friendly to encourage participation.

6. **Open-Door Policy:** Maintain an open-door policy where employees feel empowered to approach their supervisors or safety personnel with safety-related

feedback or concerns at any time. Encourage transparent communication and active listening to address issues promptly and effectively.

7. **Regular Check-ins:** Schedule regular check-ins or toolbox talks focused specifically on safety topics to provide opportunities for employees to voice their opinions, ask questions, and share feedback in a group setting. Use these sessions to reinforce the importance of safety and promote a culture of collaboration and engagement.

8. **Employee Surveys:** Administer periodic employee surveys that include questions related to safety culture, perceptions of management's commitment to safety, and opportunities for improvement. Analyze survey results to identify trends, areas of strength, and areas requiring attention.

9. **Incorporate Feedback into Decision-Making:** Actively incorporate employee feedback into decision-making processes related to safety policies, procedures, and initiatives. Demonstrate to employees that their input is valued and that their feedback contributes to positive changes within the organization.

10. **Follow-Up and Communication:** Follow up with employees who provide feedback to acknowledge their contributions and communicate any actions taken in response to their input. Provide regular updates on the status of ongoing safety improvement efforts to

demonstrate organizational commitment to addressing employee feedback.

By soliciting feedback from employees on safety practices, procedures, and attitudes, organizations can gain valuable insights, identify areas for improvement, and engage employees in the continuous enhancement of the safety culture.

4.3.3 Implementing Iterative Changes: Continuously evaluate and refine safety practices and procedures based on feedback and lessons learned, striving for continuous improvement in safety performance.

Implementing iterative changes is a fundamental aspect of fostering a culture of continuous improvement in safety performance within an organization. Here's how organizations can effectively implement iterative changes in their safety practices and procedures:

1. **Feedback Analysis:** Regularly analyze feedback collected from employees, safety incident reports, near-miss investigations, and safety audits to identify recurring themes, trends, and areas for improvement.

2. **Root Cause Analysis:** Conduct thorough root cause analyses of safety incidents and near misses to understand the underlying factors contributing to the events. Use this information to inform the development of targeted corrective actions and preventive measures.

3. **Benchmarking:** Benchmark safety performance against industry standards, best practices, and organizational goals to assess performance gaps and identify opportunities for improvement. Compare safety metrics over time to track progress and measure the effectiveness of implemented changes.

4. **Continuous Monitoring:** Implement systems for ongoing monitoring and surveillance of safety performance indicators, such as injury rates, near-miss reporting, safety compliance metrics, and leading indicators. Use real-time data to detect emerging safety issues and proactively address them.

5. **Cross-Functional Collaboration:** Foster collaboration and communication among different departments, teams, and stakeholders involved in safety management. Encourage interdisciplinary problem-solving and knowledge sharing to leverage diverse perspectives and expertise.

6. **Pilot Programs:** Pilot test new safety initiatives, procedures, or technologies on a small scale before full implementation to assess their effectiveness and identify potential challenges or unintended consequences. Solicit feedback from pilot participants to inform adjustments and improvements.

7. **Continuous Training and Education:** Provide ongoing training and education to employees at all levels of the organization on relevant safety topics, procedures, and best practices. Offer refresher courses,

toolbox talks, and skill-building workshops to reinforce safety competencies and promote a culture of continuous learning.

8. **Adaptive Response:** Be prepared to adapt and adjust safety practices and procedures in response to changing circumstances, emerging risks, or lessons learned from previous incidents. Maintain flexibility and agility in the face of evolving safety challenges and organizational needs.

9. **Leadership Support:** Secure commitment and support from organizational leadership for continuous improvement initiatives in safety. Empower safety professionals and frontline workers to drive change and innovation and allocate resources and incentives to support improvement efforts.

10. **Performance Review:** Regularly review and evaluate the effectiveness of implemented changes in safety practices and procedures. Use performance metrics, employee feedback, and other relevant data to assess outcomes, identify areas of success, and pinpoint areas requiring further attention or refinement.

By implementing iterative changes and striving for continuous improvement in safety practices and procedures, organizations can enhance their ability to prevent incidents, mitigate risks, and cultivate a culture of safety excellence.

SUMMARY OF CHAPTER 4: INTEGRATING ATTITUDE-BASED SAFETY INTO DAILY PRACTICES

In this chapter, we explore the critical aspects of embedding safety practices into the daily routines and culture of organizations.

4.1 Embedding Safety in Organizational Culture To foster a culture of safety, leadership must set the tone by modeling positive safety attitudes and behaviors. Clear expectations for safety are crucial, and organizations should communicate them consistently throughout all levels. Furthermore, creating accountability mechanisms, such as performance evaluations and recognition programs, ensures individuals are held responsible for their safety actions.

4.2 Encouraging Proactive Safety Behaviors Empowering employees to take ownership of safety is essential. By providing training, resources, and opportunities for participation in safety initiatives, organizations empower their workforce to actively engage in safety practices. Promoting observation and reporting of safety hazards and near misses encourages a proactive approach to safety. Rewarding proactive safety behaviors through incentive programs, peer recognition, and public acknowledgment reinforces the importance of safety.

4.3 Fostering Continuous Improvement Learning from incidents and near misses is a cornerstone of continuous improvement. By conducting thorough investigations and implementing corrective actions, organizations can glean valuable insights for enhancing safety practices. Soliciting feedback from employees on safety practices, procedures, and attitudes facilitates continuous improvement efforts. Implementing iterative changes based on feedback and lessons learned ensures that safety practices and procedures evolve to meet changing needs and challenges, ultimately contributing to continuous improvement in safety performance.

As we transition from Chapter 4 to Chapter 5, we move from the implementation phase to the evaluation and sustainability of Attitude-Based Safety practices. Chapter 4 emphasized the critical aspects of integrating safety into daily organizational practices, focusing on leadership's role in setting the tone, establishing clear expectations, and creating accountability mechanisms. By empowering employees, promoting proactive safety behaviors, and fostering a culture of continuous improvement, organizations can lay a strong foundation for a safety-centric culture. Now, in Chapter 5, we delve into the measurement and sustenance of these efforts, recognizing the importance of assessing safety attitudes, sustaining positive behaviors, and celebrating successes.

In Chapter 5, we explore the essential components of Measuring and Sustaining Attitude-Based Safety. We begin by discussing the importance of measuring safety attitudes through appropriate metrics and analyzing data to identify areas for improvement. By benchmarking against industry standards and organizational goals, we gain insights into performance and opportunities for enhancement. Moving forward, we explore strategies for sustaining positive attitudes, including reinforcement tactics, continuous engagement initiatives, and empowering employees through involvement and decision-making. Finally, we highlight the significance of celebrating successes, recognizing achievements, sharing success stories, and encouraging peer-to-peer recognition to reinforce a culture of safety excellence.

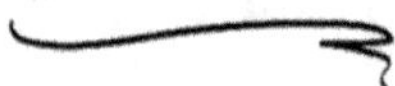

Chapter 5: Measuring and Sustaining Attitude-Based Safety

Continuous improvement is better than delayed perfection

- Mark Twain

Measuring and Sustaining Attitude-Based Safety is essential for several reasons:

1. **Evaluation and Improvement**: Measuring safety attitudes allows organizations to evaluate the effectiveness of their safety programs and initiatives. By collecting data on safety perceptions, behaviors, and attitudes, organizations can identify areas of strength and weakness, pinpointing where improvements are needed. This data-driven approach enables targeted interventions to address safety issues proactively.

2. **Risk Management**: Measuring safety attitudes helps organizations identify potential risks and hazards before they lead to accidents or incidents. By understanding employees' perceptions of safety and their willingness to adhere to safety protocols, organizations can implement preventive measures to mitigate risks and create a safer work environment.

3. **Compliance and Regulation**: Many industries are subject to regulatory requirements regarding workplace safety. Measuring safety attitudes ensures compliance

with these regulations by providing evidence of efforts to maintain a safe working environment. It also helps organizations identify gaps in compliance and take corrective actions to avoid penalties and legal repercussions.

4. **Employee Engagement and Morale**: Sustaining positive safety attitudes is crucial for maintaining high levels of employee engagement and morale. When employees feel safe and valued in the workplace, they are more motivated, productive, and committed to their work. Measuring safety attitudes allows organizations to track changes in employee perceptions over time and take proactive steps to address any issues that may arise.

5. **Continuous Improvement**: Sustaining Attitude-Based Safety requires ongoing effort and attention. By regularly measuring safety attitudes and monitoring progress, organizations can identify opportunities for continuous improvement. This iterative process enables organizations to adapt to changing circumstances, emerging risks, and evolving best practices, ensuring that safety remains a top priority in the long term.

Overall, Measuring and Sustaining Attitude-Based Safety is vital for creating a culture of safety excellence, protecting the well-being of employees, and achieving organizational success.

5.1.1 Selecting Metrics: Identify key performance indicators (KPIs) for measuring safety attitudes, such as employee surveys, observation data, and incident reports.

Selecting appropriate metrics is crucial for effectively measuring safety attitudes within an organization. Key performance indicators (KPIs) provide valuable insights into the current state of safety attitudes, helping organizations identify areas for improvement and track progress over time. Here are some common metrics for measuring safety attitudes:

1. **Employee Surveys**: Surveys are a valuable tool for gathering feedback directly from employees about their perceptions of safety in the workplace. Questions can cover various aspects, including safety culture, leadership support, communication effectiveness, and adherence to safety procedures. Analyzing survey responses allows organizations to understand employee attitudes and identify areas of concern or improvement.

2. **Observation Data**: Observation data involves systematically observing workplace activities to assess compliance with safety protocols and identify potential hazards or unsafe behaviors. By recording observations and categorizing them based on predefined criteria, organizations can track trends, identify recurring

issues, and take corrective actions to address safety concerns.

3. **Incident Reports**: Incident reports provide valuable information about safety incidents, near misses, and hazardous situations that occur in the workplace. Analyzing incident data allows organizations to identify root causes, patterns, and trends related to safety attitudes and behaviors. By understanding the factors contributing to incidents, organizations can implement preventive measures to reduce the likelihood of future occurrences.

4. **Safety Perception Surveys**: Safety perception surveys focus specifically on employees' perceptions of safety culture, leadership commitment, communication effectiveness, and other relevant factors. These surveys help organizations gauge the overall safety climate within the organization and identify areas where improvements are needed. Comparing survey results over time allows organizations to track changes in safety attitudes and assess the effectiveness of safety initiatives.

5. **Safety Compliance Metrics**: Safety compliance metrics measure the extent to which employees adhere to safety policies, procedures, and regulations. This may include metrics such as the number of safety violations, percentage of employees completing safety training, and rate of safety policy adherence. Monitoring compliance metrics helps organizations identify areas

of non-compliance and take corrective actions to improve safety attitudes and behaviors.

6. **Safety Culture Surveys**: These surveys assess employees' perceptions of the organization's safety culture, including attitudes towards safety, perceptions of leadership commitment, and overall safety climate.

7. **Near Miss Reporting Rate**: This metric tracks the number of near misses reported within a specific period, providing insights into potential hazards and opportunities for preventive action.

8. **Safety Training Completion Rate**: Measures the percentage of employees who have completed required safety training programs, indicating the organization's commitment to employee education and compliance with safety regulations.

9. **Safety Audit Findings**: Evaluates the results of safety audits or inspections to identify deficiencies, non-compliance issues, and areas for improvement in safety practices and procedures.

10. **Lost Time Injury Frequency Rate (LTIFR)**: Calculates the number of lost time injuries per million hours worked, providing a standardized measure of workplace injury severity and safety performance.

11. **Safety Compliance Score**: Assesses the organization's overall compliance with safety regulations, standards, and policies, based on audits, inspections, and regulatory requirements.

12. **Safety Perception Index**: Combines various safety perception survey results to create a comprehensive index reflecting employees' overall perceptions of safety within the organization.

13. **Safety Leadership Score**: Evaluates the effectiveness of leadership in promoting a positive safety culture and driving safety initiatives, based on leadership behaviors, communication, and visible commitment to safety.

14. **Safety Improvement Initiatives Implemented**: Tracks the number and impact of safety improvement initiatives implemented within the organization, demonstrating proactive efforts to enhance safety performance.

15. **Employee Engagement in Safety Activities**: Measures the level of employee participation and engagement in safety-related activities, such as safety meetings, safety committees, and safety initiatives, reflecting the organization's safety culture and employee involvement.

These metrics provide organizations with a comprehensive view of safety performance, helping them to identify strengths, weaknesses, and areas for improvement to drive continuous improvement in safety outcomes.

5.1.2 Analyzing Data: Analyze safety attitude data to identify trends, patterns, and areas for improvement, and use this information to inform targeted interventions.

Analyzing safety attitude data is crucial for gaining actionable insights into the organization's safety culture and identifying areas for improvement. By examining trends, patterns, and discrepancies in the data, organizations can pinpoint specific areas that require attention and develop targeted interventions to address underlying issues.

One approach to analyzing safety attitude data is to conduct a comprehensive review of survey responses, incident reports, and other relevant sources of information. This involves categorizing and organizing the data to identify common themes, such as perceptions of leadership commitment, employee engagement in safety activities, and perceptions of safety policies and procedures. By aggregating and summarizing the data, organizations can identify overarching trends and patterns that may indicate areas of strength or areas for improvement.

Another important aspect of data analysis is identifying outliers or anomalies in the data that may warrant further investigation. This could include unusually high or low scores on specific survey questions, a significant increase in the number of incident reports in a particular department, or discrepancies between different groups or locations within the organization. By digging deeper into these outliers, organizations can uncover root causes and develop targeted interventions to address underlying issues.

Overall, analyzing safety attitude data enables organizations to make informed decisions about safety initiatives and interventions, allocate resources effectively, and track progress over time. By leveraging data-driven insights, organizations can cultivate a positive safety culture, mitigate risks, and ultimately create safer and healthier work environments for employees.

Here are few additional approaches to analyze safety attitude data and visualize the findings using various charts and graphs:

1. **Comparative Analysis:** Compare safety attitude data across different groups within the organization, such as departments, shifts, or job roles. Use bar charts or radar charts to visually represent the differences in attitudes between these groups and identify areas of disparity or alignment.

2. **Time-Series Analysis:** Track changes in safety attitude data over time to identify trends and patterns. Create line charts or area charts to visualize how safety attitudes have evolved over weeks, months, or years. This analysis can help identify improvements or deterioration in safety culture and assess the impact of interventions over time.

3. **Correlation Analysis:** Explore relationships between safety attitude data and other relevant metrics, such as

injury rates, near-miss incidents, or safety compliance metrics. Use scatter plots or correlation matrices to assess the strength and direction of correlations and identify potential influencing factors.

4. **Segmentation Analysis:** Segment the workforce based on demographic variables (e.g., age, gender, tenure) or job-related factors (e.g., job role, work location) and analyze safety attitude data separately for each segment. Use stacked bar charts or grouped bar charts to compare attitudes across different segments and identify demographic or job-related factors that may influence safety perceptions.

5. **Text Mining and Sentiment Analysis:** Analyze open-ended survey responses or qualitative feedback to extract key themes and sentiments related to safety attitudes. Use word clouds or sentiment analysis tools to visualize the most frequently mentioned topics and the overall sentiment (positive, negative, or neutral) associated with safety attitudes.

6. **Benchmarking Analysis:** Compare safety attitude data against industry benchmarks or best practices to assess performance relative to peers or industry standards. Use benchmarking dashboards or spider charts to visualize how the organization's safety attitudes compare to industry norms and identify areas for improvement.

7. **Geospatial Analysis:** Analyze safety attitude data based on geographic locations or work sites to identify

regional or site-specific trends. Use heatmaps or geographic information system (GIS) tools to visualize variations in safety attitudes across different locations and prioritize interventions accordingly.

By applying these approaches and visualizing the findings using appropriate charts and graphs, organizations can gain deeper insights into safety attitudes, identify opportunities for improvement, and make data-driven decisions to enhance safety culture and performance.

5.1.3 Benchmarking and Comparison: Compare safety attitude data against industry benchmarks and organizational goals to assess performance and identify opportunities for enhancement.

Benchmarking and comparison play a crucial role in evaluating safety attitude data within an organization. By comparing this data against industry benchmarks and organizational goals, companies can gain valuable insights into their safety performance and identify areas for improvement.

Firstly, comparing safety attitude data against industry benchmarks allows organizations to assess their performance relative to their peers or industry standards. This helps in understanding where the organization stands in terms of safety culture and performance compared to others in the same sector. It also provides context for interpreting the data and identifying areas where the organization may be lagging behind or excelling.

Secondly, comparing safety attitude data against organizational goals enables companies to measure progress towards their specific safety objectives. By aligning safety attitudes with strategic goals, organizations can ensure that efforts to improve safety culture are driving tangible results and contributing to the overall success of the business. This comparison helps in identifying any gaps between current performance and desired outcomes, allowing for targeted interventions to bridge these gaps and drive continuous improvement.

Overall, benchmarking and comparison provide organizations with valuable insights and actionable information to enhance their safety culture and performance. By leveraging these comparisons, companies can benchmark themselves against industry standards, track progress towards organizational goals, and identify opportunities for enhancement to foster a safer and more productive work environment.

Imagine a Fortune 500 manufacturing company that has consistently ranked among the top performers in safety culture and performance over the past three years. By comparing its safety attitude data against industry benchmarks, such as injury rates or employee surveys, this company may have found that its recordable injury rate is significantly lower than the industry average. This indicates a strong safety culture and a proactive approach to preventing workplace accidents.

Similarly, suppose this manufacturing company sets ambitious goals to further improve its safety performance, aiming to reduce its recordable injury rate by 20% within the next three years. By regularly analyzing safety attitude data and tracking progress against these goals, the company can identify areas for improvement and implement targeted interventions. For instance, they may introduce new safety training programs, enhance hazard identification processes, or invest in advanced safety technologies to mitigate risks.

As a result of these efforts, the company sees a steady decline in recordable injuries and an increase in employee engagement with safety initiatives. This positive trend not only enhances the company's reputation as a safe workplace but also contributes to improved productivity and morale among employees. By benchmarking its safety performance against industry standards and organizational goals, this Fortune 500 company continues to sustain and enhance its safety culture, setting a benchmark for others to follow.

5.2 SUSTAINING POSITIVE ATTITUDES

5.2.1 Reinforcement Strategies: Implement strategies for reinforcing positive safety attitudes and behaviors, such as recognition programs, positive feedback, and leadership support.

Sustaining positive attitudes towards safety requires ongoing reinforcement to ensure that employees remain engaged and committed to safety principles. One effective strategy is to implement reinforcement programs aimed at recognizing and rewarding positive safety attitudes and behaviors. This can include:

Recognition Programs: Establishing formal recognition programs to acknowledge individuals or teams who demonstrate exemplary safety attitudes and behaviors. This could involve monthly or quarterly awards ceremonies where employees are publicly recognized for their contributions to safety.

Positive Feedback: Providing regular, constructive feedback to employees who exhibit positive safety attitudes and behaviors. This feedback should be specific, timely, and focused on reinforcing desired behaviors, such as wearing appropriate PPE or reporting safety concerns.

Leadership Support: Ensuring that leadership actively supports and reinforces positive safety attitudes throughout the organization. Leaders can demonstrate their commitment to safety by participating in safety activities, visibly promoting safety initiatives, and regularly communicating the importance of safety to all employees.

Peer Recognition: Encouraging peer-to-peer recognition of positive safety behaviors within teams or departments. This can foster a culture of accountability and support, where employees feel empowered to recognize and appreciate their colleagues' contributions to safety.

Incentive Programs: Implementing incentive programs that reward employees for achieving safety milestones or targets. This could include bonuses, gift cards, or other tangible rewards for individuals or teams who consistently demonstrate safe behaviors and contribute to a positive safety culture.

Safety Culture Surveys: Conducting regular safety culture surveys to gather feedback from employees about their perceptions of safety within the organization. This provides valuable insights into areas where reinforcement may be needed and helps identify opportunities for improvement.

Safety Committees: Establishing safety committees comprised of representatives from various departments or teams to provide input on safety initiatives and promote a collaborative approach to safety improvement efforts. Involving employees in decision-making processes fosters a sense of ownership and engagement.

Continuous Training and Development: Offering ongoing training and development opportunities related to safety to keep employees informed about best practices, regulatory updates, and emerging risks. Investing in employee education demonstrates the organization's commitment to safety and empowers individuals to make informed decisions.

Safety Audits and Inspections: Conducting regular safety audits and inspections to identify potential hazards, assess compliance with safety protocols, and ensure that corrective actions are implemented in a timely manner. Providing feedback from audits and inspections helps reinforce the importance of adherence to safety standards.

Safety Communication Channels: Establishing open communication channels, such as safety suggestion boxes, anonymous reporting systems, or safety hotlines, to encourage employees to voice their safety concerns and suggestions for improvement. Ensuring that employees feel heard and valued promotes a culture of transparency and trust.

By incorporating these reinforcement strategies into their safety programs, organizations can further enhance their ability to sustain positive attitudes towards safety and drive continuous improvement in safety performance.

Re-engineering strategies can also play a crucial role in reinforcing positive safety attitudes and behaviors within an organization, as stated below:

1. **Process Optimization**: Re-engineering safety processes and procedures to make them more efficient, effective, and user-friendly can positively impact safety attitudes. When safety protocols are streamlined and optimized, employees are more likely to adhere to them consistently, leading to a safer work environment overall.

2. **Technology Integration**: Leveraging technology to enhance safety initiatives can reinforce positive behaviors. For example, implementing digital safety management systems or mobile applications that facilitate incident reporting, safety training, and real-time communication can empower employees to actively engage in safety practices and contribute to a culture of safety.

3. **Data-Driven Decision Making**: Utilizing data analytics and performance metrics to identify areas for improvement and inform safety reinforcement strategies can be highly effective. By analyzing safety data trends and patterns, organizations can pinpoint areas of concern, target interventions where they are most needed, and track progress over time to ensure sustained positive outcomes.

4. **Continuous Improvement**: Applying principles of continuous improvement to safety processes through re-engineering efforts ensures that safety initiatives remain dynamic and responsive to changing needs and challenges. By regularly reviewing and refining safety protocols based on feedback and lessons learned, organizations can continuously reinforce positive safety attitudes and behaviors.

5. **Cross-Functional Collaboration**: Engaging cross-functional teams in the re-engineering process fosters a sense of ownership and collective responsibility for safety. By involving employees from various departments in the redesign of safety processes and procedures, organizations can ensure that safety reinforcement strategies are tailored to meet the unique needs and perspectives of different workgroups.

Overall, re-engineering strategies can serve as powerful tools for reinforcing positive safety attitudes and behaviors by optimizing processes, leveraging technology, utilizing data insights, fostering continuous improvement, and promoting cross-functional collaboration in pursuit of a safer workplace.

5.2.2 Continuous Engagement: Keep safety on the forefront of employees' minds through ongoing communication, training, and engagement initiatives.

Continuous engagement is vital for maintaining a strong safety culture within an organization. Here's how it can be illustrated:

1. **Regular Safety Communication**: Implementing regular safety communication channels ensures that safety remains a top priority for employees. This can include safety newsletters, emails, bulletin boards, or digital signage displaying safety messages and reminders throughout the workplace. By keeping safety information visible and accessible, employees are reminded of the importance of safe practices on a consistent basis.

2. **Ongoing Training Programs**: Providing continuous safety training and education reinforces positive safety behaviors and equips employees with the knowledge and skills needed to identify and mitigate risks. Offering a variety of training formats, such as in-person workshops, online courses, toolbox talks, and hands-on simulations, ensures that training remains engaging and relevant to employees' roles and responsibilities.

3. **Engagement Initiatives**: Implementing engagement initiatives that encourage active participation in safety activities fosters a sense of ownership and accountability among employees. This can include safety committees or task forces where employees collaborate to identify safety issues, develop solutions, and implement improvements. Recognition programs that celebrate safety milestones, achievements, and contributions also promote a positive safety culture and encourage continued engagement.

4. **Feedback Mechanisms**: Establishing feedback mechanisms allows employees to voice their concerns, suggestions, and ideas related to safety. This can be done through anonymous suggestion boxes, safety suggestion programs, or regular safety meetings where employees are encouraged to share their feedback openly. Actively listening to employee feedback demonstrates that their input is valued and helps identify areas for improvement in safety practices and procedures.

5. **Leadership Visibility and Support**: Demonstrating leadership visibility and support for safety initiatives reinforces the importance of safety throughout the organization. Leaders can actively participate in safety activities, communicate safety expectations, and recognize employees for their safety contributions. By leading by example, leaders set a positive tone for safety and inspire greater engagement and commitment from employees at all levels.

Overall, continuous engagement in safety through communication, training, engagement initiatives, feedback mechanisms, and leadership support helps to keep safety at the forefront of employees' minds and fosters a culture of safety excellence within the organization.

These outcomes get reflected in reports of several leading auditing firms through organizational culture, risk management, and compliance. Some of these firms include:

1. **Deloitte**: Deloitte's risk advisory services often cover safety culture, risk management, and compliance strategies. Their reports may provide insights into best practices for embedding safety into organizational culture and sustaining positive attitudes towards safety.

2. **PricewaterhouseCoopers (PwC)**: PwC offers risk assurance and compliance services that may include assessments of safety culture and performance. Their reports could provide valuable insights into measuring safety attitudes, benchmarking against industry standards, and implementing reinforcement strategies.

3. **KPMG**: KPMG's risk consulting services encompass various aspects of safety management, including culture assessment, compliance monitoring, and performance improvement. Their reports may offer insights into effective engagement strategies, leadership support, and continuous improvement initiatives.

4. **EY (Ernst & Young)**: EY provides risk advisory services that cover safety culture assessments, safety management systems, and regulatory compliance. Their reports may offer guidance on measuring safety attitudes, identifying areas for enhancement, and sustaining positive safety behaviors.

5. **Bureau Veritas**: As a leading testing, inspection, and certification company, Bureau Veritas offers services related to safety management and compliance auditing. Their reports may focus on best practices for integrating safety into daily practices, measuring safety performance, and achieving continuous improvement.

These auditing firms often publish thought leadership articles, whitepapers, and industry insights on their websites, which can be valuable resources for organizations seeking to enhance their safety culture and practices. Additionally, they may offer customized consulting services to address specific safety challenges and opportunities within organizations.

5.2.3 Empowerment and Involvement: Empower employees to actively participate in safety initiatives and decision-making processes, fostering a sense of ownership and commitment to safety.

Empowerment and involvement are crucial aspects of fostering a strong safety culture within an organization. By empowering employees to actively participate in safety initiatives and decision-making processes, organizations can tap into their collective knowledge and expertise, thereby fostering a sense of ownership and commitment to safety among employees.

One way to empower employees is by involving them in safety committees or task forces dedicated to identifying and addressing safety concerns. These committees can provide a platform for employees to voice their opinions, share their experiences, and contribute ideas for improving safety practices. Additionally, organizations can empower employees by providing them with the necessary training, resources, and support to take on leadership roles in safety initiatives. By giving employees, a voice and a stake in safety-related decisions, organizations can create a culture where safety is everyone's responsibility, leading to improved safety outcomes and a safer work environment overall.

Participation and involvement

Participation in various safety activities not only increases employees' interest in safety but also encourages them to take initiatives to improve safety standards within the organization. When employees actively participate in safety-related activities such as safety committees, hazard identification, safety training sessions, and safety drills, they become more engaged and invested in safety practices.

Participation provides employees with firsthand experience and exposure to safety issues, helping them better understand the importance of safety and the potential risks involved in their work environment. As employees become more involved, they are more likely to take ownership of safety initiatives and suggest improvements to existing safety protocols. This increased interest and engagement can lead to the development of innovative safety solutions and the implementation of best practices to enhance safety standards across the organization.

Furthermore, participation in safety activities fosters a culture of collaboration and teamwork, where employees feel empowered to contribute their ideas and expertise to improve safety outcomes. This collective effort not only strengthens the organization's safety culture but also builds trust and camaraderie among employees, ultimately creating a safer and more productive work environment.

5.3 CELEBRATING SUCCESSES

5.3.1 Recognizing Achievements: Celebrate milestones and achievements in safety performance through formal recognition events, awards ceremonies, and public acknowledgments.

Recognizing achievements in safety performance is vital for fostering a culture of safety excellence within an organization. By celebrating milestones and accomplishments, organizations reinforce positive safety behaviors and attitudes, motivating employees to continue prioritizing safety in their daily work. Here are some keyways in which recognizing achievements contributes to enhancing attitude-based safety:

1. **Acknowledgment of Efforts:** Recognizing achievements acknowledges the efforts and dedication of individuals and teams towards improving safety

outcomes. This acknowledgment validates their commitment to safety and reinforces the importance of their contributions to the organization's overall safety culture.

2. **Inspiration and Motivation:** Celebrating milestones and achievements inspires and motivates others by showcasing examples of success in safety performance. When employees see their colleagues being recognized for their efforts, it serves as a powerful motivator for them to emulate similar behaviors and strive for excellence in safety.

3. **Reinforcement of Safety Values:** Formal recognition events and awards ceremonies reinforce safety as a core organizational value. By publicly acknowledging and celebrating safety achievements, organizations demonstrate their commitment to prioritizing safety and creating a safe work environment for all employees.

4. **Boosting Morale and Engagement:** Recognition and acknowledgment of achievements boost employee morale and engagement by making them feel valued and appreciated for their contributions. This positive reinforcement enhances job satisfaction and strengthens employee commitment to safety initiatives.

5. **Catalyst for Continuous Improvement:** Celebrating achievements encourages a culture of continuous improvement by highlighting successes and identifying areas for further enhancement. By

recognizing milestones and accomplishments, organizations motivate employees to continue striving for safety excellence and actively participate in ongoing improvement efforts.

In summary, recognizing achievements in safety performance is a powerful tool for reinforcing positive safety behaviors and attitudes, inspiring employees, and fostering a culture of safety excellence. By celebrating milestones and accomplishments, organizations not only acknowledge the efforts of their workforce but also reinforce the importance of safety as a shared responsibility and core organizational value.

5.3.2 Sharing Success Stories: Share success stories and best practices in safety attitudes and behaviors to inspire and motivate employees and reinforce positive safety culture.

Sharing success stories is a powerful way to reinforce positive safety attitudes and behaviors within an organization. By highlighting real-life examples of successful safety initiatives, employees are inspired and motivated to emulate those behaviors, leading to a stronger safety culture. Here's how sharing success stories contributes to enhancing safety attitudes:

1. **Inspiration and Motivation:** Success stories serve as tangible examples of what can be achieved through dedication to safety. When employees hear about their colleagues' achievements in promoting safety, they are inspired to take similar actions and strive for excellence in their own safety practices. These stories provide a

sense of motivation by demonstrating that safety goals are attainable and worth pursuing.

2. **Learning Opportunities:** Success stories offer valuable learning opportunities for employees to glean insights and best practices from their peers. By sharing details about the strategies, techniques, and interventions that led to successful safety outcomes, employees can learn from each other's experiences and apply those lessons to their own work environments. This knowledge-sharing fosters a culture of continuous improvement where employees actively contribute to enhancing safety practices.

3. **Positive Reinforcement:** Sharing success stories reinforces positive safety behaviors by recognizing and celebrating achievements. When individuals or teams are publicly acknowledged for their contributions to safety, it reinforces the importance of those behaviors and encourages others to follow suit. Positive reinforcement creates a ripple effect throughout the organization, where employees feel valued for their commitment to safety and are motivated to maintain and exceed those standards.

4. **Cultural Norms:** Success stories help to establish and reinforce cultural norms around safety within the organization. By consistently sharing examples of safety excellence, organizations communicate their commitment to prioritizing safety and create expectations for similar behaviors across all levels and

departments. Over time, these stories become ingrained in the organizational culture, shaping attitudes and behaviors towards safety as a core value.

Overall, sharing success stories plays a crucial role in nurturing a positive safety culture by inspiring, educating, and reinforcing desired behaviors. By leveraging the power of storytelling, organizations can create a shared narrative of safety success that drives continuous improvement and fosters a collective commitment to safety excellence.

5.3.3 Encouraging Peer-to-Peer Recognition: Encourage employees to recognize and celebrate each other's contributions to safety through peer-to-peer recognition programs and initiatives.

Encouraging peer-to-peer recognition in safety initiatives is a powerful strategy to foster a culture of appreciation, collaboration, and accountability within an organization. Here's how it contributes to enhancing safety attitudes:

1. **Promotes Positive Relationships:** Peer-to-peer recognition strengthens interpersonal relationships among employees by fostering a culture of appreciation and mutual respect. When colleagues acknowledge and celebrate each other's contributions to safety, it creates a supportive environment where individuals feel valued and respected for their efforts. This positive reinforcement strengthens team cohesion and encourages collaboration towards common safety goals.

2. **Drives Accountability:** Peer-to-peer recognition holds individuals accountable for their safety behaviors and encourages them to take ownership of safety outcomes. When employees actively recognize and commend their peers for adhering to safety protocols, it reinforces the importance of safety standards and encourages adherence to best practices. This sense of accountability motivates employees to maintain high safety standards and reinforces a collective commitment to safety excellence.

3. **Strengthens Trust and Communication:** Peer-to-peer recognition enhances trust and communication within teams by promoting open dialogue and feedback exchange. When employees feel empowered to acknowledge and celebrate safety achievements among their peers, it fosters a culture of transparency and communication. This open exchange of recognition builds trust among team members and facilitates constructive discussions around safety improvements and challenges.

4. **Boosts Morale and Engagement:** Peer-to-peer recognition boosts employee morale and engagement by fostering a positive work environment where achievements are celebrated and appreciated. When employees receive recognition from their peers for their safety efforts, it enhances their sense of job satisfaction and motivation. This positive reinforcement of safety behaviors contributes to higher levels of engagement and commitment to organizational safety goals.

5. **Sustains Positive Safety Culture:** Peer-to-peer recognition contributes to the sustainability of a positive safety culture by reinforcing desired behaviors and attitudes over time. When recognition becomes ingrained in the organizational culture, it becomes a natural part of daily interactions among employees. This sustained focus on safety recognition reinforces the organization's commitment to safety excellence and helps embed safety as a core value within the workplace.

Overall, encouraging peer-to-peer recognition in safety initiatives empowers employees to actively participate in promoting a safe work environment. By fostering a culture of appreciation, accountability, and collaboration, peer-to-peer recognition strengthens safety attitudes and behaviors, driving continuous improvement in safety performance.

SUMMARY OF CHAPTER 5: MEASURING AND SUSTAINING ATTITUDE-BASED SAFETY

5.1 Measuring Safety Attitudes In this section, the focus is on measuring safety attitudes through various metrics:

- **Selecting Metrics:** Key performance indicators (KPIs) such as employee surveys, observation data, and incident reports are identified to gauge safety attitudes.

- **Analyzing Data:** Safety attitude data is analyzed to discern trends, patterns, and areas for improvement, enabling targeted interventions.

- **Benchmarking and Comparison:** Safety attitude data is compared against industry benchmarks and organizational goals to evaluate performance and identify opportunities for enhancement.

5.2 Sustaining Positive Attitudes This section delves into sustaining positive safety attitudes through effective strategies:

- **Reinforcement Strategies:** Strategies like recognition programs, positive feedback, and leadership support are implemented to reinforce positive safety behaviors.

- **Continuous Engagement:** Safety is kept at the forefront of employees' minds through ongoing communication, training, and engagement initiatives.

- **Empowerment and Involvement:** Employees are empowered to actively participate in safety initiatives and decision-making processes, fostering a sense of ownership and commitment to safety.

5.3 Celebrating Successes The focus here is on celebrating safety successes to reinforce positive safety culture:

- **Recognizing Achievements:** Milestones and achievements in safety performance are celebrated through formal recognition events, awards ceremonies, and public acknowledgments.

- **Sharing Success Stories:** Success stories and best practices in safety attitudes and behaviors are shared to inspire and motivate employees, reinforcing positive safety culture.

- **Encouraging Peer-to-Peer Recognition:** Employees are encouraged to recognize and celebrate each other's contributions to safety through peer-to-peer recognition programs and initiatives, fostering a culture of appreciation and collaboration.

Conclusion

As we conclude this comprehensive journey through "Attitude-Based Safety: Cultivating a Culture of Safety Through Positive Attitudes," it is clear that fostering a safe and resilient environment goes beyond mere adherence to protocols. It requires a profound shift in attitudes and behaviors at every level of an organization. From understanding the foundational role of attitude in safety to developing positive safety attitudes and overcoming barriers, each chapter has underscored the necessity of embedding safety into the very fabric of organizational culture. Leaders play a pivotal role in setting the tone, establishing clear expectations, and creating accountability, while employees must be empowered and encouraged to engage proactively in safety practices.

Chapter 5, "Measuring and Sustaining Attitude-Based Safety," emphasized the importance of continuous evaluation and reinforcement of positive safety attitudes. By selecting the right metrics, analyzing data, and benchmarking performance, organizations can identify areas for improvement and sustain a high level of safety culture. Reinforcement strategies, continuous engagement, and celebrating successes are crucial for maintaining a strong safety attitude. As you reflect on the insights gained from this book, I encourage you to embrace your unique logical brain, empower yourself and others, and continue exploring and developing attitudes that contribute to a safe and accident-free environment. The journey of cultivating a positive safety culture is ongoing, and with commitment and perseverance, we can create workplaces where safety is ingrained in every action and decision.

1. Understanding Attitude-Based Safety

- **The Power of Attitude in Safety:** Positive attitudes significantly impact safety outcomes. Real-life examples demonstrate how attitudes influence safety behaviors and overall workplace safety.

- **Attitude Formation and Maintenance:** Attitudes towards safety are shaped by past experiences, social influences, and organizational culture. Consistent reinforcement and education are crucial for maintaining positive safety attitudes.

- **Attitude as the Core Factor:** Attitudes form the foundation of effective safety programs. Aligning organizational values with a commitment to safety and empowering individuals can drive significant safety improvements.

2. Developing Positive Safety Attitudes

- **Promoting Safety Awareness:** Creating a culture of safety awareness involves training, communication, and leveraging technology. Engaging employees in safety initiatives is vital.

- **Building a Culture of Responsibility:** Establishing clear safety expectations and fostering peer support and accountability encourages a sense of responsibility for safety.

- **Leadership's Influence on Attitudes:** Leadership plays a critical role in modeling and promoting positive safety attitudes. Training leaders to prioritize safety can transform organizational safety culture.

3. Overcoming Attitude Barriers

- **Addressing Resistance to Change:** Understanding and effectively communicating the reasons for safety changes can mitigate resistance and increase acceptance.

- **Changing Negative Attitudes:** Providing education, support, and opportunities for self-reflection can help individuals shift from negative to positive safety attitudes.

- **Cultivating Resilience:** Building mental toughness and promoting work-life balance are essential for fostering resilience and maintaining positive attitudes towards safety.

4. Integrating Attitude-Based Safety into Daily Practices

- **Embedding Safety in Organizational Culture:** Leadership sets the tone for safety culture. Clear expectations and accountability mechanisms are essential for integrating safety into daily practices.

- **Encouraging Proactive Safety Behaviors:** Empowering employees to take ownership of safety, promoting observation and reporting, and rewarding proactive behaviors are key strategies.

- **Fostering Continuous Improvement:** Learning from incidents, soliciting feedback, and implementing iterative changes drive continuous safety improvements.

5. Measuring and Sustaining Attitude-Based Safety

- **Measuring Safety Attitudes:** Identifying and analyzing key performance indicators (KPIs) helps monitor and improve safety attitudes. Benchmarking against industry standards aids in assessing performance.

- **Sustaining Positive Attitudes:** Reinforcement strategies, continuous engagement, and empowering employees ensure the sustainability of positive safety attitudes.

- **Celebrating Successes:** Recognizing achievements, sharing success stories, and encouraging peer-to-peer recognition enhance safety culture and morale.

Encouraging Readers to Continue Exploring and Developing Their Attitude and Behavior to Stay Safe

Cultivating a safety culture rooted in positive attitudes is an ongoing journey. By embracing the insights and strategies discussed in this book, readers can continue to explore and develop their attitudes and behaviors, contributing to a safer and more resilient work environment. Continuous learning, engagement, and empowerment are essential for sustaining these positive changes.

The Journey of Continuous Improvement:

Cultivating a culture of safety is not a one-time effort but a continuous journey. It requires persistent exploration, development, and reinforcement of positive attitudes and behaviors. By actively engaging in this ongoing process, individuals and organizations can foster a safer, more resilient work environment.

1. Embrace Lifelong Learning: Safety is an evolving field, and staying informed about the latest best practices, technologies, and research is essential. Encourage readers to:

- Attend workshops, seminars, and training sessions on safety.

- Subscribe to safety journals, newsletters, and online platforms that offer up-to-date information and resources.

- Participate in professional safety organizations and networks to share knowledge and experiences with peers.

2. Self-Reflection and Personal Growth: Personal attitudes and behaviors significantly influence safety outcomes. Readers should be encouraged to:

- Regularly reflect on their attitudes towards safety and identify areas for improvement.

- Set personal safety goals and track progress towards achieving them.

- Seek feedback from colleagues and supervisors to gain insights into their safety behaviors and attitudes.

3. Engage in Open Communication: Open communication is vital for continuous improvement in safety attitudes and behaviors. Readers can:

- Foster a culture of openness where safety concerns and suggestions can be discussed without fear of retribution.

- Participate in safety meetings, forums, and discussions to share experiences and learn from others.

- Encourage a two-way dialogue between employees and management to ensure everyone's voice is heard and valued.

4. Lead by Example: Leadership is crucial in promoting and sustaining a positive safety culture. Readers in leadership positions can:

- Model positive safety attitudes and behaviors for their teams.

- Recognize and reward employees who demonstrate a strong commitment to safety.

- Provide mentorship and support to help others develop their safety attitudes and behaviors.

5. Empower and Involve Others: Empowering employees to take ownership of safety can drive significant improvements. Encourage readers to:

- Involve employees in safety initiatives and decision-making processes.

- Provide opportunities for employees to lead safety projects and initiatives.

- Create peer-to-peer recognition programs to celebrate contributions to safety.

6. Utilize Technology and Innovation: Leveraging technology can enhance safety practices and awareness. Readers should explore:

- Utilizing mobile apps and digital platforms for real-time safety reporting and communication.

- Implementing virtual reality simulations for safety training and hazard recognition.

- Using data analytics to monitor safety performance and identify trends and areas for improvement.

7. Celebrate Successes: Recognizing and celebrating achievements in safety can reinforce positive behaviors and attitudes. Encourage readers to:

- Celebrate milestones and successes through formal events, awards, and public acknowledgments.

- Share success stories and best practices within the organization to inspire and motivate others.

- Encourage peer-to-peer recognition to build a supportive and collaborative safety culture.

8. Foster a Resilient Mindset: Building resilience helps individuals and organizations adapt to challenges and maintain a strong commitment to safety. Readers can:

- Promote mental health and well-being programs to support resilience.

- Encourage work-life balance to reduce stress and enhance focus on safety.

- Develop coping strategies and provide support for employees facing challenges.

By continuing to explore and develop their attitudes and behaviors towards safety, readers can contribute to a dynamic and proactive safety culture. This ongoing commitment to learning, self-improvement, and collaboration will not only enhance safety performance but also create a work environment where everyone feels valued, respected, and safe.

Empowering readers to embrace their unique logical brain to enhance positive safe attitude.

Every individual has the potential to contribute to a culture of safety through their attitudes and behaviors. By leveraging their unique logical thinking, readers can critically assess safety practices, identify areas for improvement, and drive positive change. Empowerment and ownership of safety initiatives at all levels are crucial for achieving a resilient and accident-free environment.

Harnessing the Power of Logic and Reason:

One of the core messages of "Attitude-Based Safety: Cultivating a Culture of Safety Through Positive Attitudes" is the importance of using our logical brain to enhance safety attitudes and behaviors. By understanding and leveraging the power of logic and reason, readers can make more informed decisions, solve problems more effectively, and create a safer work environment.

1. Critical Thinking: Encouraging readers to apply critical thinking skills to safety scenarios can lead to better decision-making and problem-solving. Readers can:

- Analyze potential hazards logically and assess the risks involved.

- Evaluate safety protocols and procedures to identify areas for improvement.

- Make data-driven decisions to enhance safety practices.

2. Evidence-Based Approaches: Readers should be encouraged to use evidence and data to guide their safety attitudes and behaviors. They can:

- Collect and analyze data on safety incidents and near misses to identify patterns and root causes.

- Use research and case studies to learn about successful safety interventions and best practices.

- Implement changes based on empirical evidence rather than assumptions or anecdotal information.

3. Logical Problem-Solving: Empowering readers to approach safety challenges with a logical problem-solving mindset can lead to innovative solutions. Readers can:

- Break down complex safety issues into manageable components to address each aspect effectively.

- Use logical frameworks, such as root cause analysis or the 5 Whys technique, to identify underlying issues.

- Develop and test hypotheses to find the most effective solutions to safety problems.

4. Structured Training Programs: Readers can benefit from structured training programs that focus on developing logical reasoning and analytical skills. Organizations can:

- Provide training on critical thinking, data analysis, and problem-solving as part of their safety programs.

- Use simulations and scenario-based training to allow employees to practice applying logical reasoning to real-world safety challenges.

- Encourage continuous learning and professional development to keep skills sharp and up to date.

5. Encouraging Scientific Thinking: Promoting a scientific approach to safety can help readers develop a rational and evidence-based attitude. Readers can:

- Conduct experiments and pilot programs to test new safety interventions.

- Encourage a culture of inquiry where questions are welcomed, and curiosity is rewarded.

- Use the scientific method to systematically investigate and solve safety-related problems.

Outcome of the Book

By the end of "Attitude-Based Safety: Cultivating a Culture of Safety Through Positive Attitudes," readers will gain a comprehensive understanding of the importance of positive safety attitudes and the role of logical thinking in enhancing safety performance. They will be equipped with practical tools and strategies to foster a proactive safety culture within their organizations.

Key Outcomes Include:

1. Improved Safety Awareness: Readers will have a heightened awareness of the impact of attitudes on safety and the importance of maintaining a positive safety culture. They will be able to recognize and address negative attitudes that may hinder safety efforts.

2. Enhanced Problem-Solving Skills: Through the application of logical reasoning and evidence-based approaches, readers will be better equipped to identify and address safety issues effectively. They will be able to implement solutions that are grounded in data and research.

3. Stronger Organizational Culture: Organizations that embrace the principles outlined in this book will benefit from a stronger, more cohesive safety culture. Employees at all levels will feel empowered to take ownership of their safety attitudes and behaviors, leading to a more engaged and committed workforce.

4. Continuous Improvement: The book encourages a mindset of continuous learning and improvement. Readers will be motivated to seek out new information, stay updated on best practices, and continuously refine their safety strategies to achieve better outcomes.

5. Practical Tools and Strategies: Readers will have access to a range of practical tools and strategies that they can implement in their workplaces to foster positive safety attitudes and behaviors. These tools will help them create a safer, more resilient work environment.

By embracing their unique logical brains and applying the concepts from this book, readers can make significant strides in enhancing their safety attitudes and behaviors, ultimately contributing to a safer and more productive workplace.

Scope for Further Research and Development

While "Attitude-Based Safety: Cultivating a Culture of Safety Through Positive Attitudes" explores various aspects of safety attitudes and practices, it merely scratches the surface of this complex and evolving field. The topics and solutions presented serve as foundational elements, offering a springboard for ongoing exploration and innovation.

Expanding Understanding of Safety Attitudes: The interplay between attitudes and safety behaviors is multifaceted and dynamic. Further research can explore how different variables—such as cultural diversity, generational differences, and psychological factors—impact safety attitudes. Longitudinal studies could also provide insights into how these attitudes evolve over time and under different organizational conditions.

Innovative Training Methods: Developing and testing new training methods that effectively shape positive safety attitudes remains a critical area for research. This could include the use of virtual reality, gamification, and other interactive technologies to create immersive learning experiences that resonate with employees.

Advanced Data Analytics: Harnessing the power of advanced data analytics and machine learning can lead to more sophisticated methods for measuring and predicting safety attitudes and behaviors. Research in this area can help develop predictive models that identify potential safety risks before they manifest, allowing for proactive interventions.

Psychological and Social Dynamics: Further investigation into the psychological and social dynamics that influence safety attitudes can yield deeper insights. This includes studying the impact of leadership styles, peer influence, and social networks within organizations on safety behaviors.

Tailored Interventions: Research can also focus on designing and testing tailored interventions that address specific organizational contexts and individual differences. Personalized approaches to safety training and communication may prove more effective than one-size-fits-all solutions.

Policy and Regulatory Implications: Exploring the implications of safety attitudes for policy and regulatory frameworks can inform better governance and compliance strategies. This includes examining how regulatory requirements influence organizational safety cultures and identifying best practices for policy implementation.

Global Perspectives: Comparative studies across different countries and industries can provide a global perspective on safety attitudes and practices. Understanding the cultural nuances and industry-specific challenges can lead to the development of more universally applicable safety strategies.

Technological Integration: The integration of emerging technologies such as the Internet of Things (IoT), artificial intelligence (AI), and wearable devices in safety management systems offers another promising research avenue. These technologies can provide real-time monitoring and feedback, enhancing the effectiveness of safety interventions.

Long-Term Impact Studies: Conducting long-term impact studies to assess the sustainability and effectiveness of attitude-based safety interventions over extended periods can provide valuable insights. These studies can help refine and improve strategies to ensure they deliver lasting benefits.

Cross-Disciplinary Approaches: Collaborative research that brings together insights from psychology, organizational behavior, engineering, and other disciplines can foster innovative solutions. Cross-disciplinary approaches can help develop comprehensive strategies that address the multifaceted nature of safety attitudes.

In conclusion, while this book provides a solid foundation, the field of attitude-based safety is ripe with opportunities for further research and development. By continuing to explore, innovate, and refine our understanding and practices, we can make significant strides towards creating safer and more resilient work environments.

May I request a review?

Could I kindly ask for your consideration to leave a review on the publisher's platform for the book?

I hope you've found the book engaging and insightful on this captivating subject. While reviews might carry less weight for established authors, they hold immense value for writers like me who are emerging and lack a significant following.

Your review could be instrumental in drawing more readers to my work, inspiring them to explore my books.

As you immerse yourself in the content of this book, I believe you'll be inclined to share your thoughts in a review.

Writing your sentiments about the book will require just a brief two minutes of your time. Your support and engagement mean a lot to me, and I'm eager to see your review on the publisher's page.

Your reviews contribute to the dialogue and feedback from readers, fostering a greater connection between authors and their audience.

I assure you, taking just a couple of minutes to share your thoughts on the book would be greatly appreciated. Your words hold the power to inspire and propel my passion for writing even further.

Thank you from the bottom of my heart for supporting my work. I eagerly await your review on the publisher page, where your words will resonate and touch the hearts of fellow readers.

Happy reading and heartfelt gratitude.

Disclaimer

Information shared through this book about the power of pure intention is based on our personal understanding, knowledge, and belief and appears to be reliable, as we have learned from different authorities and personal experiences in our lives.

Some information is taken from reliable sources, but this is not expected to replace any professional medical advice given on specific conditions. Readers should consult a qualified expert before making any decisions based on the information presented.

The author and publisher cannot be held responsible for any errors or omissions in the information presented in this book. Readers are encouraged to make their own judgement and seek professional advice when necessary.

This disclaimer applies to any harm or damage, or any action carried out due to follow-up of the suggestions contained herein while remaining engaged in many complex issues of life.

As you read this book, you agree to learn and accept all risks generally on the implementation of suggestions contained herein. The content of this book is for informational purposes only.

The use of this book implies your acceptance of this disclaimer. We cannot guarantee the level of success you may experience by following the suggestions contained in this book, although these are generally applicable to many people, and highly beneficial for varied fields of activities.

About the Author

Dr. Gurudas Bandyopadhyay brings a unique blend of academic expertise and extensive professional experience to his book "Attitude-Based Safety." With a Doctorate in Philosophy from the Indian Institute of Technology, Kharagpur, specializing in HRM, and postgraduate qualifications in Business Administration, Marketing Management, and Hospital Administration, Dr. Bandyopadhyay is well-equipped to provide insightful perspectives on safety management.

His career spans various esteemed organizations such as Larsen & Toubro, Haldia Petrochemicals Limited, ICI India Ltd., and Heavy Engineering Corporation Ltd., where he held key roles in safety, health, and environment management. Dr. Bandyopadhyay's experience as a Fire & Safety Officer, Chief Manager in Safety, and HSE Advisor underscores his deep understanding of safety practices across diverse industries.

In addition to his professional endeavors, Dr. Bandyopadhyay has made significant contributions to academia, serving as Director of Post Graduate Studies and Dean & Associate Vice President (Academic) at reputed institutions. His academic qualifications, including a membership examination in Fire Engineering from IFE, UK and a Diploma in Industrial Safety, further enrich his expertise in safety management. He is Fellow Member (Life Member) in IFE India and Emeritus member of American Society of Safety Professionals.

With his comprehensive understanding of safety principles, coupled with his academic background and hands-on experience, Dr. Bandyopadhyay's book promises to offer readers valuable insights into cultivating positive safety attitudes and fostering a culture of safety in various organizational contexts.

More books from the author

Name of Book	Relinks.me
Dream And Dare Series (DAD)	
Atomic Thoughts	https://relinks.me/B08Q8KQ8NH
Self-Care Power	https://relinks.me/B08TT4SRNQ
Magic of Dreaming Bigger	https://relinks.me/B097MDRQGK
Enjoy Living Each Day	https://relinks.me/B09CKJ7CGL
Brain Energy Source	https://relinks.me/B0BTDYVZ6P
Be Younger Forever	https://relinks.me/B0BW512L5K
The Power Of Pure Intention	https://relinks.me/B0CK67CCY3
Empower Your Thoughts	https://relinks.me/B0CQFYVL87
Health And Happiness Series (HAH)	
Master Healthy Eating Habits	https://relinks.me/B0BQXMVNBF
10 Easy Steps to GOOD HEALTH	https://relinks.me/B07MJ3VFLF

Be Happy Be You	https://relinks.me/B09MTDK498
Be Your Mental Health Therapist	https://relinks.me/B0C4M8GKC4
Fitness – 10 Essential Steps to A Healthier You	https://relinks.me/B0C9RQCL77
The Relationship Code	https://relinks.me/B0CRVY18DQ
Lifestyle And Safety (LAS)	
Care For SAFE ATTITUDE	**https://relinks.me/B08271HLY3**
Positive Living Made Simple	https://relinks.me/B0CD4K3P4N
The Power Of Self-Discipline	https://relinks.me/B0CGSJ9GZ5
Harmony Through Indian Heritage	https://relinks.me/B0CS9MHGMC
Art of Incremental Growth	https://relinks.me/B0CW1H2PHV
Success And Prosperity (SAP)	
Try Again Today	https://relinks.me/B09WN2H9YB
Mental Toughness for adults	https://relinks.me/B09YTTT5P2

Awaken The CREATIVE Giant Within	https://relinks.me/B0B69J3RQD
The Breakthrough Code	https://relinks.me/B0BMHVDCHP
Strive And Thrive	https://relinks.me/B0C5V7HNST
The Idea Catalyst	https://relinks.me/B0CGKDL3GB
The Art of Everyday Assertiveness	https://relinks.me/B0CM36SBKH
Transform 2 Triumph (TTT)	
Break The Cycle Of Poverty	https://relinks.me/B0CWDVJFKF
Overcoming adversity: Stories of Triumph	https://relinks.me/B0D3253L83
Redefine Social Welfare: A Blueprint for Change	https://relinks.me/B0D3ZMQLJP
Redefine Social Welfare: Workbook	https://relinks.me/B0D3ZQ2DD1
Master Your Superpower	https://relinks.me/B0D5FYFR39

The Upcoming Book

"The Psychology of Safety: *From Attitudes to Habits*"

The book is a comprehensive guide to transforming safety attitudes into ingrained habits, revolutionizing safety culture in industries and communities. With a blend of psychological insights, practical strategies, and real-world examples, this book equips readers with the tools to foster positive safety behaviors and create lasting change.

From understanding the role of attitudes in safety to implementing lifestyle changes for unconscious safety, each chapter explores key concepts and offers actionable steps for improvement.

Dr. Bandyopadhyay delves into behavioral psychology theories, habit formation techniques, and leadership strategies, providing a roadmap for cultivating a culture of safety that permeates every aspect of life.

With a focus on continuous improvement and empowerment, "The Psychology of Safety" challenges readers to rethink their approach to safety and take proactive steps towards creating safer environments.

Whether you're a safety professional, organizational leader, or concerned individual, this book offers invaluable insights and inspiration for driving positive change and making safety a top priority.

7 key benefits from the book to readers

Deep Understanding of Safety Psychology: Readers will gain a profound understanding of the psychological factors that influence safety attitudes and behaviors, enabling them to approach safety initiatives with greater insight and effectiveness.

Practical Strategies for Behavior Change: The book provides practical strategies and techniques for translating positive safety attitudes into actionable behaviors, empowering readers to implement tangible changes in their personal and professional lives.

Habit Formation Techniques: With a focus on habit formation, readers will learn proven techniques for developing and reinforcing safe habits, making safety practices second nature and sustainable in the long term.

Leadership Insights: Dr. Bandyopadhyay offers valuable insights into the role of leadership in promoting a culture of safety, equipping readers with the knowledge and tools to lead by example and inspire others to prioritize safety.

Empowerment and Accountability: Through discussions on empowerment and accountability, readers will discover how to empower individuals and communities to take ownership of their safety, fostering a collective responsibility for creating safe environments.

Continuous Improvement: The book emphasizes the importance of continuous improvement in safety practices, providing guidance on how to adapt and evolve safety initiatives to meet changing needs and challenges.

Measurable Results: By identifying key metrics and indicators for assessing safety performance, readers will learn how to measure the success of their safety initiatives and celebrate achievements, driving motivation and momentum for further improvement.

To connect with the author

Website:

https://drgurudas.com

YouTube Channel:

https://www.youtube.com/channel/UCXMr5UUXEDTKg aV8Jq3lSmw

Facebook Page:

https://www.facebook.com/HolisticHealthHappinessPros perity

LinkedIn:

https://www.linkedin.com/in/gurudas-bandyopadhyay-75b30220/

Instagram:

https://www.instagram.com/healthyhappyprosperous/

ConvertKit:

https://winning-thinker-8854.ck.page/92cd3161e1

Acknowledgment

I would like to acknowledge the support received from various people and organizations with whom I was associated for considerable time and who have contributed a lot to develop my knowledge base, starting from school and service life; whose collective wisdom has illuminated the path toward empowered thinking.

I would prefer first to express my deep heartfelt gratitude to my grandfather who was also a renowned spiritual teacher, Professor Hara Govinda Smriti Ratna. He was the founder Professor of Anandamayee Chattuspathi. He used to teach me tsocietyIndian texts and to live in harmony with society and environment.

I am grateful to my parents, other senior family members, relatives and teachers for their blessings and for giving me the inspiration, courage and total support to continue higher studies and sharing lessons.

I thank my wife and children for supporting me always to write books to share my thoughts to help the aspiring adults.

I am grateful to the eminent authors whose books I read and learn a lot, whose videos I watch and gain lot of knowledge to share with others.

I am grateful to be inspired by Google scholar, various websites, ChatGPT, TEDx Talks, YouTube and such other sites for enriching my knowledge base.

I am deeply grateful for the support and inspiration from Author Freedom Hub Mentor Mr. Som Bathla and fellow authors, which have fueled the creation of this book.

I am thankful to the readers and audiences for showing interest in my articles, books and educational videos. Their feedback and enthusiasm have motivated me to continue exploring the profound concepts of intentional thinking and attraction.

Additional resources for readers

Important references to learn more about the subjects of safety psychology, behavior-based safety, habit formation, and cultivating a safety culture. These are only indicative. All the courses and books and journals may not be available now, but you may get something and find something useful with these resources.

A) Books:

"The Power of Habit: Why We Do What We Do in Life and Business" by Charles Duhigg

"Safe by Accident? Take the Luck out of Safety: Leadership Practices that Build a Sustainable Safety Culture" by Judy L. Agnew and Aubrey C. Daniels

"Drive: The Surprising Truth About What Motivates Us" by Daniel H. Pink

"Safety Differently: Human Factors for a New Era" by Sidney Dekker

"Safety-I and Safety-II: The Past and Future of Safety Management" by Erik Hollnagel

"Mindfulness for Beginners: Reclaiming the Present Moment—and Your Life" by Jon Kabat-Zinn

"Nudge: Improving Decisions About Health, Wealth, and Happiness" by Richard H. Thaler and Cass R. Sunstein

"Grit: The Power of Passion and Perseverance" by Angela Duckworth

"The Checklist Manifesto: How to Get Things Right" by Atul Gawande

"Thinking, Fast and Slow" by Daniel Kahneman

"Blink: The Power of Thinking Without Thinking" by Malcolm Gladwell

"Switch: How to Change Things When Change Is Hard" by Chip Heath and Dan Heath

"Behavior-Based Safety Process: Managing Involvement for an Injury-Free Culture" by Thomas R. Krause

"Leading with Safety" by Thomas R. Krause

"Safety Culture: An Innovative Leadership Approach" by Nathan Crutchfield and James Roughton

"The Behavior-Based Safety Guide: Implementing and Managing a Successful BBS Program" by Terry E. McSween

"Quality Safety Edge: The Role of Quality and Behavioral Science in Safety Performance" by Terry L. Mathis and Shawn M. Galloway

"Proven Strategies in Behavioral Safety" by Timothy D. Ludwig

"People-Based Safety: The Source" by E. Scott Geller

"Behavioral Safety: Theory, Method and Application" edited by Tim Marsh and David T. Hoyle

"From Accidents to Zero: A Practical Guide to Improving Your Workplace Safety Culture" by Andrew Sharman

"Behavior-Based Safety in Organizations: Current Approaches and Future Directions" edited by Richard H. Ginnett and Kevin P. McCarty

B) Research Articles and Papers:

"Behavior-Based Safety and Occupational Risk Management" by E. Scott Geller

"The Role of Attitudes in Safety Management" by Yorio, Mittlemark, and Dembe

"Motivational Factors in Safety Compliance: A Meta-Analysis of Empirical Evidence" by Neal and Griffin

"A Review of the Literature on Near Miss Reporting" by Phimister, Oktem, Kleindorfer, and Kunreuther

C) Online Resources:

National Safety Council (NSC)

Website: NSC

Provides a wealth of resources, research, and guidelines on various aspects of safety, including workplace safety, road safety, and home safety.

Occupational Safety and Health Administration (OSHA)

Website: OSHA

Offers regulations, safety guidelines, and resources for improving workplace safety.

Centers for Disease Control and Prevention (CDC) - National Institute for Occupational Safety and Health (NIOSH)

Website: NIOSH

Provides research and information on workplace safety and health.

Behavioral Science Technology (BST)

Website: BST

Focuses on behavior-based safety and offers resources, training, and consultancy services.

D) Other Websites

American Society of Safety Professionals (ASSP)

Website: ASSP https://www.assp.org/

Provides resources, standards, and professional development for safety professionals.

National Institute for Occupational Safety and Health (NIOSH)

Website: NIOSH

Offers research and guidelines for workplace safety and health.

International Association of Safety Professionals (IASP)

Website: IASP

Focuses on the development and promotion of safety management practices globally.

Safety and Health Magazine

Website: Safety and Health Magazine

Publishes news, research, and resources on occupational safety and health.

Centers for Disease Control and Prevention (CDC) - Workplace Safety and Health

Website: CDC Workplace Safety

Provides resources for promoting health and safety in the workplace.

Scientific Committee on Occupational Health in Construction Industry https://scohici.org/

Safety Engineers Association:

https://safetyengineersassociation.org/

E) Journals:

Journal of Safety Research

Publishes original research on all aspects of safety, including behavior-based safety, safety culture, and risk management.

Safety Science

A multidisciplinary journal covering research on the science and practice of safety, including human behavior, safety management systems, and accident analysis.

These references provide a comprehensive foundation for understanding and implementing the principles on safety psychology, behavior-based safety, and habit formation.

"The Effects of Behavior-Based Safety Interventions on Safety Behavior: A Meta-Analysis" by Tomás Ruiz-Frutos, et al.

Journal: Safety Science, 2018.

Reviews the effectiveness of behavior-based safety interventions.

"Safety Culture and Safety Performance in Construction Industry: The Mediating Role of Safety Knowledge and Motivation" by Samah Boutrous and Peter T. McCabe

Journal: Safety Science, 2019.

Examines the relationship between safety culture and performance in the construction industry.

"Mindfulness and Safety Performance in a High-Risk Industry" by Jon Kabat-Zinn and Saki F. Santorelli

Journal: Journal of Occupational Health Psychology, 2020.

Studies the impact of mindfulness practices on safety performance in high-risk environments.

These references will provide a comprehensive foundation for understanding and applying the concepts of safety psychology, behavior-based safety, and habit formation in various contexts.

F) TED Talks:

"The Surprising Science of Happiness" by Dan Gilbert

Insights into how we perceive risk and make decisions that impact safety.

"What Makes Us Feel Good About Our Work?" by Dan Ariely

Discusses motivation and its relevance to safe work behavior.

"The Power of Vulnerability" by Brené Brown

Explores the role of vulnerability and trust in creating a culture of safety.

G) YouTube Videos:

"Behavior-Based Safety Overview" by E. Scott Geller

An introduction to behavior-based safety by a leading expert in the field.

"Safety Culture: The Essential Elements" by SafetyCulture

Discusses the key components of building a strong safety culture.

"Understanding Human Error" by Sidney Dekker

Dekker provides insights into human error and safety management.

H) Podcasts:

"Safety on Tap" by Andrew Barrett

Covers various topics on safety leadership, culture, and improvement.

"The Safety of Work" by Dr. David Provan and Dr. Drew Rae

Discusses the latest research and concepts in occupational safety.

"Safety Consultant with Sheldon Primus"

Provides insights and tips for safety professionals.

I) Online Platforms:

LinkedIn Learning:

LinkedIn Learning offers courses on various aspects of safety, including safety leadership, risk management, and behavior-based safety. You can find courses taught by industry experts and practitioners.

Udemy:

Udemy has a wide range of courses on safety-related topics, including behavior-based safety, safety culture, and occupational health. These courses are often created by professionals with practical experience in the field.

Coursera:

Coursera partners with universities and institutions to offer online courses on safety management, workplace safety, and related subjects. You can find courses that cover behavior-based safety principles and applications.

American Society of Safety Professionals (ASSP):

ASSP offers online training courses and webinars on various safety topics, including behavior-based safety, safety management systems, and risk assessment. These courses are developed by safety professionals and experts in the field.

National Safety Council (NSC):

The NSC provides online training programs and resources for workplace safety, including courses on behavior-based safety and safety leadership. These courses are designed to help organizations improve safety performance.

J) Courses in Udemy in this concern

On Udemy, you can find several courses related to safety psychology, behavior-based safety (BBS), and related topics. Here are some examples of courses you might find on Udemy:

"Behavior Based Safety (BBS) Awareness"

This course introduces behavior-based safety principles and practices, covering topics such as identifying unsafe behaviors, implementing observation programs, and creating a safety culture.

"Safety Leadership: The 6 Vital Behaviors"

This course focuses on the leadership aspects of safety, teaching participants how to lead and inspire safety initiatives in their organizations. Topics include communication, accountability, and coaching for safety.

"Occupational Health and Safety (OHS) Fundamentals"

This course covers the fundamentals of occupational health and safety, including risk assessment, hazard identification, and regulatory compliance. It provides a broad overview of safety management principles.

"Safety Culture: Building a High-Performance Workplace"

This course explores the concept of safety culture and how organizations can create and sustain a positive safety culture. Topics include leadership, employee engagement, and continuous improvement.

"Safety Management Systems (SMS) Fundamentals"

This course provides an overview of safety management systems, including their components, implementation, and effectiveness. It covers topics such as policy development, risk assessment, and incident investigation.

"Introduction to Industrial Hygiene"

This course introduces participants to the principles of industrial hygiene, including exposure assessment, hazard control, and regulatory requirements. It is suitable for professionals working in occupational health and safety.

"Ergonomics: Designing for People"

This course focuses on ergonomic principles and their application in workplace design and management. Topics include ergonomic risk factors, workstation setup, and injury prevention.

"Incident Investigation: A Practical Guide"

This course teaches participants how to conduct effective incident investigations, including root cause analysis, corrective action planning, and reporting. It is suitable for safety professionals and managers.

These are just a few examples of the types of courses you can find on Udemy related to safety psychology, behavior-based safety, and occupational health and safety. But read the course descriptions, reviews, and instructor profiles to find the best courses for your learning needs and interests.

K) EdX and Coursera:

Both edX and Coursera offer a variety of courses related to safety psychology, behavior-based safety (BBS), and occupational health and safety. Here are some examples of courses you might find on these platforms: However, these are indicative and many courses might have closed now, bringing up new ones.

edX:

"Occupational Health in Developing Countries" by the University of Bergen

This course explores occupational health issues in developing countries, including workplace hazards, risk assessment, and preventive measures.

"Occupational Health in Developing Countries" by the University of Bergen

This course explores occupational health issues in developing countries, including workplace hazards, risk assessment, and preventive measures.

"Occupational Safety and Health in Construction" by the University of Manchester

This course focuses on safety management in the construction industry, covering topics such as hazard identification, risk assessment, and regulatory compliance.

"Safety and Health in the Construction Industry" by Delft University of Technology

This course provides an overview of safety and health management in the construction industry, including safety culture, safety leadership, and accident prevention.

"Managing Occupational Health and Safety" by the University of Toronto

This course covers the principles and practices of occupational health and safety management, including risk assessment, hazard control, and regulatory compliance.

Coursera:

"Workplace Safety and Health" by the University of Washington

This course provides an introduction to workplace safety and health, covering topics such as hazard identification, risk assessment, and injury prevention.

"Occupational Health in Developing Countries" by the University of Bergen

This course explores occupational health issues in developing countries, including workplace hazards, risk assessment, and preventive measures.

"Occupational Safety and Health in Construction" by the University of Manchester

This course focuses on safety management in the construction industry, covering topics such as hazard identification, risk assessment, and regulatory compliance.

"Workplace Safety and Health Leadership" by the University of California, Irvine

This course teaches participants how to lead and manage workplace safety and health programs, including safety culture, safety leadership, and employee engagement.

"Safety and Health Management" by the University of Illinois at Urbana-Champaign

This course covers the principles and practices of safety and health management, including risk assessment, hazard control, and regulatory compliance.

These are just a few examples of the courses available on edX and Coursera related to safety psychology, behavior-based safety, and occupational health and safety.

L) Courses like "Lead Auditor courses" ISO 14000, 18000, 9001, and others

10 more ISO standards, each representing a different area of management system:

ISO 27001 - Information Security Management System (ISMS):

ISO 27001 specifies requirements for establishing, implementing, maintaining, and continually improving an information security management system within the context of the organization's overall business risks.

ISO 22000 - Food Safety Management System (FSMS):

ISO 22000 sets out the requirements for a food safety management system and can be applied by any organization in the food chain, from primary producers to food manufacturers, transport, and storage operators, and retail and food service outlets.

ISO 50001 - Energy Management System (EnMS):

ISO 50001 provides requirements for establishing, implementing, maintaining, and improving an energy management system, aimed at enabling organizations to follow a systematic approach to achieve continual improvement of energy performance.

ISO 45001 - Occupational Health and Safety Management System (OH&SMS):

ISO 45001 specifies requirements for an occupational health and safety management system, providing a framework for organizations to improve employee safety, reduce workplace risks, and create better working conditions.

ISO 26000 - Social Responsibility:

ISO 26000 provides guidance on social responsibility, helping organizations integrate social, environmental, ethical, and governance considerations into their operations and strategies.

ISO 13485 - Medical Devices Quality Management System (QMS):

ISO 13485 specifies requirements for a quality management system for organizations involved in the design, development, production, installation, and servicing of medical devices.

ISO 31000 - Risk Management:

ISO 31000 provides principles, framework, and guidelines for managing risks effectively, assisting organizations in identifying, assessing, and managing risks to achieve their objectives.

ISO 9004 - Quality Management - Quality of an Organization:

ISO 9004 provides guidance for organizations to enhance their overall performance and achieve sustained success through the effective application of a quality management approach.

ISO 22301 - Business Continuity Management System (BCMS):

ISO 22301 specifies requirements for establishing, implementing, maintaining, and continually improving a business continuity management system, enabling organizations to prepare for and respond to disruptive incidents.

ISO 14064 - Greenhouse Gas Management and Accounting:

ISO 14064 provides standards for quantifying, monitoring, reporting, and verifying greenhouse gas emissions and removals, helping organizations manage and mitigate their carbon footprint.

These ISO standards cover a diverse range of management system areas, enabling organizations to address various aspects of their operations, including quality, safety, environmental performance, information security, and social responsibility.

M) Other Standards & Guidelines

In addition to ISO standards, there are various standards, guidelines, and regulations issued by government organizations, national safety councils, the World Health Organization (WHO), and other international bodies. These standards and guidelines often focus on specific industries, sectors, or areas of concern. Here are some examples:

Government Organizations:

OSHA Standards (USA):

The Occupational Safety and Health Administration (OSHA) sets and enforces standards to ensure safe and healthy working conditions for workers in the United States.

HSE Regulations (UK):

The Health and Safety Executive (HSE) in the United Kingdom develops and enforces regulations to protect workers' health and safety.

CCOHS Guidelines (Canada):

The Canadian Centre for Occupational Health and Safety (CCOHS) provides guidelines and resources to promote health and safety in Canadian workplaces.

Ministry of Labour Standards (Various Countries):

Ministries of Labour in different countries often establish standards and regulations related to workplace safety, health, and labor rights.

National Safety Councils:

National Safety Council (NSC - USA):

The NSC provides resources, training, and advocacy to promote safety in various areas, including workplaces, roads, and homes.

British Safety Council (BSC - UK):

The BSC offers training, qualifications, and advisory services to improve health, safety, and environmental management in workplaces.

Australian Safety Council (Australia):

The Australian Safety Council provides information, training, and accreditation services to enhance safety and health outcomes in Australia.

World Health Organization (WHO):

WHO Guidelines on Occupational Health:

The WHO develops guidelines and recommendations to protect workers' health and promote occupational health and safety worldwide.

WHO International Health Regulations (IHR):

The IHR is a legal instrument binding on 196 countries to prevent, protect against, control, and provide a public health response to the international spread of diseases.

Other International Bodies:

International Labour Organization (ILO):

The ILO develops international labor standards, including conventions and recommendations related to occupational safety and health, employment, and labor rights.

European Agency for Safety and Health at Work (EU-OSHA):

EU-OSHA provides information, tools, and resources to improve occupational safety and health across European Union member states.

International Organization for Standardization (ISO):

Apart from ISO management system standards, ISO also develops technical standards in various areas, including occupational health and safety, environmental management, and quality management.

These standards, guidelines, and regulations complement ISO standards and provide additional frameworks and requirements to address specific safety, health, and environmental concerns at national and international levels. Organizations can use a combination of these standards and guidelines to enhance their safety management systems and meet regulatory requirements.

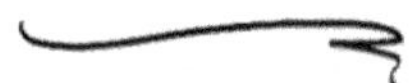